NO PLACE FOR AUTISM?

Jaime Hoerricks, PhD

NO PLACE FOR AUTISM?

Exploring the solitary forager hypothesis of autism in light of place identity

The Disability Studies Collection

Collection editors
**Dr Damian Mellifont &
Dr Jen Smith-Merry**

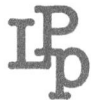

LᴘP
p

First published in 2023 by Lived Places Publishing.

British Library Cataloguing in Publication Data
A CIP record for this book is available from the British Library

ISBN: 9781915271815 (pbk)
ISBN: 9781915271839 (ePDF)
ISBN: 9781915271822 (ePUB)

Cover design by Fiachra McCarthy
Book design by Rachel Trolove of Twin Trail Design
Typeset by Newgen Publishing UK

Lived Places Publishing
Long Island
New York 11789

www.livedplacespublishing.com

Abstract

Guided from a lived experience point of view, *No place for autism?* explores how what we consider to be autism can vary from place to place. Is it a disability? If it is a disability, what is the better model for framing the authentic autistic experience: the medical model, the social model, or the ecological-enactive model of disability? If it is simply a difference in the human experience, what about structural supports and accommodations? The answers might surprise you.

Working from the premise that the autistic system is the result of 50,000 years of natural selection, the author posits that the autistic system works as designed and then unpacks the design in a highly detailed fashion, diving deep into questions of autistic identity across time and place. Noting that autism is both a set of traits and an identity, implications of this design-centric approach are given from the standpoint of place. That is to say, are there places and spaces where one might feel more or less disabled? If so, why… and what can be done to give **place** to autistic people and autistic communities?

Keywords

Asperger's Disorder; Autism Spectrum Disorder (ASD); autistic; disability studies; neurodivergent; special education; teaching studies

Contents

1
Introduction

Learning objective

Students will be able to synthesize the lived experience of autistic adults in the context of place, based upon the supplied descriptions and related research.

Activity

At the end of the chapter, students will engage in an activity that explores the evolution of their intersectional identities as their place or context has changed over time.

Key vocabulary, terms, references, and background knowledge-building resources

You will find explanations of key vocabulary and terms at the end of each chapter, together with the chapter's references and knowledge-building resources.

Meet the author

Hello and welcome. My name is Jaime Hoerricks, the author of this text. I'll be your facilitator through this experience. I happen to be autistic and non-verbal. I don't just mention this in passing. It is an important factor in this text. You see, for many years the greater autistic community has asked that future work focus on those areas that improve autistic people's day-to-day lives. Also, that there needs to be more involvement from autistic people in autism research, as well as the creation and publication of materials that deal with autism. This work is an attempt to do just that – to feature the work of an autistic researcher and educator with a diverse range of lived experiences. These experiences reinforce the central premise of this text, that how one experiences autism can vary depending upon one's intersecting identities as well as one's place on this planet.

Allow me to explain. As I write this, I'm over 50 years old and living in the rural mountains of northern Los Angeles County, California. My experience of being autistic thus spans times when autism wasn't widely recognized in the world to the present, where we are again questioning what it means to be autistic. I was originally diagnosed in 2012 with Sensory Processing Disorder and Sensory Integration Disorder (both related to my confused processing of incoming sensory information), and Asperger's Disorder (related to my processing of the world). With the change from DSM-IV-TR to DSM-5, these individual diagnoses were changed within the medical records system of my health care provider to the single diagnosis of Autism Spectrum Disorder (ASD). Like many autistic people, I have many other health issues – also known as co-morbidities. For example, I am alexithymic and histamine intolerant, which has a profound impact on how I experience the social world. Alexithymia is not only an inability to accurately describe how one feels, but an inability to correctly attribute the source of those feelings. For a hyper-empathic person, one who is constantly absorbing the feelings and energy from around them, this can be quite problematic. I'll share more on this later in the book.

Academically, I have bachelor's and master's degrees in Organizational Leadership, a master's degree in Education Instructional Design, a master's degree in Special Education, and a PhD in Education. My dissertation focused on the sensory environments on university campuses in the US that are so hostile to the autistic system that more than 60 percent of first-year autistic students voluntarily withdraw in their first semester. From the resulting data, I suggested four easy-to-accomplish tasks that college administrations could do to improve outcomes for this vulnerable population of learners. I was able to accomplish these academic achievements after learning to work in the English language in my late twenties. As a non-verbal autistic person growing up in a culturally diverse part of an English-speaking country, I did not acquire a verbal language as a child.

As a child and a young adult, I used echolalia to communicate vocally. I had a very low success rate with the dozen or so words and phrases I had memorized. I lived in a working-class suburb of migrants who largely came from northern and eastern Europe, Mexico, and Armenia. Thus, my basket of phrases contained a range of languages, which further complicated my language development. German, making more sense to me than English, was the first language that I attempted to learn. It helped that I had German-speaking friends who were largely supportive of my efforts.

I managed to graduate from high school in the top 25 of my class of almost 500 students despite being functionally illiterate. This fact has been the largest factor informing my decision to become an educator. But first, I had to learn to operate in the world of the verbal.

As my ability to process verbal language developed in my late twenties, I found work as a forensic scientist. Later, after tasking my autistic brain to turn my new vocation into my special interest, I wrote a book on the uses of Photoshop for digital multimedia forensic science as a giant info-dump. It became a best-seller and is still available for sale almost 15 years after its initial publication. As I dove deep into my new special interest, I developed hyper-specialized courses around the topics in that field. These were info-dumps full of complex, hands-on exercises. Requests to host these courses took me all over the world, teaching students from over 40 countries. Then, the COVID-19 pandemic happened and shut down in-person training. With my college and professional experience around creating and facilitating engaging learning events, I transitioned into a similar career, one that the government deemed more essential than adult professional development. I enrolled in a local college's teacher preparation program and am now a credentialed special education teacher and literacy specialist.

Despite this seemingly busy blur of a schedule, I've found the time to be married for 25 years. I am a parent to an array of neurodivergent children. Through it all, our family has found a way to accommodate each other's autism, ADHD, anxiety, and OCD. Being a parent of neurodivergent children, I understand and can empathize with the Autism Parent™ movement. Yet, I don't identify within that space as the Autism Parent™ is often a neurotypical person seeking help in understanding and supporting their neurodivergent child/children. From their publications and advocacy, they don't seem to realize that their autistic child did not occur by chance, that autism is part of their family's genetic history. This movement features excessive and harmful treatments (Millman, 2020), as well as harmful "cures" (Zadrozny, 2019). That's not where me and my family are in our advocacy or identity work.

That is the 10,000-foot view of a well-lived life spent living and working across three continents. With this in mind, however, there is a saying within the American autistic community, "if you've met one autistic, you've met one autistic." This is to say, every autistic person is unique, with unique strengths and challenges. There is always a problem when someone attempts to frame something as complex as autism within their own unique experiences. This book won't attempt to do that. Instead, it will utilize multiple frameworks to illustrate, and help you investigate, how the experience of autism changes according to time, place, and identity.

Indeed, so much has been written about the autistic experience. The current trends seem to divide the work into two main silos: strengths-based memoirs or deficits-based examinations – seemingly in constant conflict with each other. Academia tends toward deficits-based pathological examination, diving into the differences between autistic people and the neurotypical, and suggesting so-called therapies or interventions to help autistics fit into a largely neurotypical world. The autistic community tends toward featuring our strengths, almost to the point of seeming to attempt to justify our existence. Some of it is co-opted by the neurotypical community and ends up as inspiration porn.

Often lost in the discussion is the relatively unpopular opinion in academic circles that what we now call autism is not new and that it has been around for quite some time. As an example, I can examine the traits and behaviors of my relatives going back generations and find so many similarities to my own experiences in the here and now. Some, like the University of Southern California's Jared Reser, even posit that these traits can be traced far back in the human genetic record.

If you've never heard of Jared Reser, you're not alone. Though the trend is starting to slowly shift in a more helpful direction, most of the current research on autism begins with the premise that the autistic brain and system are a disordered "normal" system, and then works from there to commercialize some "cure" or "treatment" (Stenson, 2019). Not so with Reser. He takes a dispassionate, non-commercial view of autism and dives deep into humanity's genetic past to examine a rather simple premise – what evolutionary forces were at work in the creation of what we now call autism and how did it survive through natural selection? In his paper on the subject (Reser, 2011), he notes that the cognitive differences currently associated with autism spectrum disorder are clear and well documented; however, modern social and occupational practices may hide their evolutionary or adaptive benefits. From an anthropological or historic perspective, he notes, the society we live in now is very different from the environment of human evolutionary adaptedness. In other words, place has quite a lot to do with our experience of autism and our ability to pass this genetic material from one generation to the next.

Yes, that's quite a mouthful. But it's a simple premise that Reser pursues, and he does so from several angles. His Solitary Forager Hypothesis builds upon his Animal Theory of Autism. Both combine to inform some of the more fundamental aspects of what we now call autism spectrum disorder. One of the subplots of his work deals with the "why autistics wander away" question, which he explores from several vantage points – hence the solitary forager name.

Along the same line, an examination of the etymology of the word autism finds that it was derived from the Greek word *autos* or self. Thus, it literally means "selfism." It's important to note that this selfism does not imply being selfish. Neither does it imply a departure from reality. We autistics often create a world which buffers us from our often-extreme sensitivities. We think and feel quite deeply (Gernsbacher and Yergeau, 2019). We struggle to fit into the neurotypical world. This selfism often results in isolation, alienation even, from our peers. We long for deep and meaningful interactions in a world where such interactions are quite often superficial. Society sees the communication of autistics as one sided or focused on our own special interests without equal sharing. But this interpretation is often influenced by identity and place. Autistic-to-autistic communication does not need to conform to the norms or desires of the neurotypical world, and thus usually doesn't.

I can relate to the solitary forager theme. I'm autistic and I've been wandering off for as long as I can recall. My most stark childhood memory of wandering off was in primary school. The "official family memory" of the event was that I missed the bus and went home with a classmate to play with him at his house. This is certainly a "just the facts" type of account. But, in the days before awareness of autism, there was no other way to explain my rather willful behavior. Willful in that it wasn't an accident; I wasn't abducted. I simply wandered off or roamed away to explore something or someone of interest. My classmate made an offer that the solitary forager in me couldn't refuse. It is a strong and lasting memory because of how it ended for me... a rather public beating for the high crime of worrying my parents by disappearing. I suspect that a swift beating has resulted for autistics of my generation wandering off and worrying their parents. Although beating children is completely out of favor in modern times, it did serve as a conditioning event. My unconscious solitary foraging tendencies needed another way to satisfy their desires (Hoerricks, 2022).

Reser's theory notes that we autistics are wired for a solitary life. He added the foraging aspects into his theory because, again, this neurotype has been around since before the time when *Homo sapiens* was slugging it out with Neanderthal, at least 50,000 years ago. The solitary wandering or roaming thus fulfills a vital biological function – we wander away from the pack to make our own way. Hunger and thirst refine our intelligent, systematizing mind toward being able to sustain our solitary desires.

But what are we foraging for in modern times? I think that part of the theory becomes unique to each autistic individual and their place in this world. That's where Glasser's Choice Theory comes in. According to Choice Theory, at all times, we're seeking to fulfill one or more of five basic needs in pursuit of our Quality World. That Quality World is our idealized life, the world as we see it, or a kind of flow state in which we have our basic needs completely met.

My next childhood memory relating to this topic is a visit by my grandmother's brother when I was six. My mother and her family are from Canada, and my great-uncle Sandy was an engineer for Ford Motors in Canada. At the point where we met, he was traveling North America testifying in trials related to crashes of certain Ford vehicles. This was 1976. It was also the day I was introduced to the concept that a professional baseball team could be created out of thin air (yes, I'm still a Toronto Blue Jays fan to this day). What Uncle Sandy placed into my consciousness was the idea that one could be paid, and paid well, to wander. That one's foraging activities could be sponsored by someone who wanted services that I could provide. This was a hint at my later career in forensics, and a roaming of the world teaching this new science.

Growing up in the lower echelons of the trade-unionist working class, my family didn't have much material wealth in comparison to those with whom I went to school. What we did have was hard earned and treasured. I say this in relation to my first bicycle. About the time I got my first bike, I was old enough to be permitted to wander farther away from the house. If I was home by a certain hour, I could roam quite far away on my bike. I explored the depth and breadth of my city. I was in no way honest with my parents about where or how far I'd gone on any particular day. In contrast to modern parents of autistic children, I was encouraged to get out of the house and stay out until the day's end. I took advantage of this freedom and pushed its limits each day.

This is also the time when I staged a series of disciplinary situations to get kicked off the school bus so I could wander my way to school. Certainly, there were bullies on the bus who were brutal in their daily assaults. But I could have easily dispatched them, as I had done to a few classmates previously. I was head and shoulders above my classmates in size. Nevertheless, I didn't want to be on the bus. The sensory assault notwithstanding, getting off the bus meant having to make my way to the school on my own… about 3 miles away. There was a set of railroad tracks that made the route even more of an adventure. So, finding out what it would take to get kicked off the bus permanently was a win-win goal for me. Soon enough, I was off the bus and walking and biking to school.

In high school, my involvement in sports also supported my wandering. Having to stay in shape for multiple sports, I got on my bike and hit the streets daily. One summer had me at the Converse All Stars basketball league. This time, I was riding my bike about 20 miles to a distant community college to play 3 hours of basketball only to bike the 20 miles home at the end. Needless to say, engaging my solitary wandering in this way led to me being in phenomenal physical shape.

This desire to wander would also appear when I was playing varsity basketball but also wanting to wrestle. In high school in the US, these sports happen in the same season. I couldn't play basketball and wrestle at the same time at the same school. So, I got on my bike once again. I snuck out after basketball practice to wrestle at the local Greco club, which met in the evenings at the local college. Again, the 5-mile bike ride through the hills after a full basketball practice only to engage in a full wrestling practice and then bike back the 5 miles led to me preserving that physique.

Unfortunately, not being aware of the context of these wanderings has led to some rather unfortunate episodes. I wandered off to college after high school, taking the first offer that came my way. My desire to leave home was greater than any advice given to me that it wasn't a good idea or that it wouldn't end well. It didn't. I wasn't ready to be fully on my own, but there I was. I even had access to a car. Boy did I ever wander. I wandered so far one Friday, and my flow state was so intense, that I missed my football game on Saturday. I completely forgot that I was in school to play football and that they owned the rights to my time. The following Monday, my coaches let me know who was in charge. The resulting behavioral conditioning event, forced fitness drills until I collapsed due to severe exhaustion, ensured that it didn't happen that way again.

Several injuries, and several unfortunate incidents later, football was over for a time, and I was wandering north to continue my education in a more supportive setting. This time I was in northern California. There, in the care of a wonderful woman who is still a dear, albeit distant, friend, I was completely on my own and able to wander in some incredible spaces. I took every advantage. So great was my desire to explore, so poor was my health relative to my autistic system, and the fact that I was functionally illiterate, it took me four years to complete the first two years of college. I didn't do well academically, still struggling as I was with language.

It was there I met the mother of my oldest son. In retrospect, she enjoyed the wandering and was keen to join in. An incredibly intelligent and resourceful woman, she was the perfect partner for me at the time, and we willingly joined forces… a rarity for the solitary type (though Reser does account for this). She had wandered so far away to California and was anxious to get back to where her heart remained, Germany. A year or so later, we had wandered across the width of the US and were exploring western Europe. It was within this space that I experienced many meltdowns as well as my first two autistic shutdowns. They scared us both tremendously. Nothing like that, the shutdowns, had ever happened to me. I had no words for what I was experiencing then. Now, I can try to put them into words that neurotypicals may understand.

Meltdowns

In children, meltdowns often present as a total loss of control with screaming, violence, spitting, and smashing things co-occurring. A child may present one or all of these behaviors while melting down. For most adults, meltdowns look different. When you're an autistic adult, particularly one who has masked well into adulthood and received a late diagnosis, you've often learned strategies to cope and not react in a visible way. It's not generally socially acceptable for an adult to throw a tantrum. Perhaps you haven't learned to cope, but you've learned to contain those urges and react in a different way to the overwhelming build-up of whatever causes your meltdowns. What do meltdowns look like for many autistic adults? Overwhelming, devastating emotion. This can manifest by crying to the point where we physically shake and can't breathe properly. Preceding this, we can have irritability, a short fuse, or we can zone out. Then there's the impatience. The getting muddled when we try to do the simplest of tasks. General forgetfulness and ineptitude moves into a complete lack of executive functioning. We can have a "don't touch me!" feeling. Next come the "don't talk to me," "leave me alone", and "I am DONE!" feelings. As this is happening, our already poor spatial awareness worsens. Adding to the problems, panic/anxiety attacks are frequently experienced along with meltdowns.

When an autistic person can't manage their meltdown and return to a calmer state, or if they're not able to manage these over longer periods of time, shutdowns will occur. It's worth noting here that medication is not helpful when dealing with meltdowns. The system simply needs a safe and calm space in which to settle down.

Shutdowns

An autistic shutdown is a freeze response as a reaction to something that has happened. It can be caused by overstimulation, a stressful situation, last-minute changes, being emotionally overwhelmed, sadness, and more. It is like a fight/flight response. During a shutdown, we can become less vocal or completely non-speaking. We can look "spaced-out" or detached from what's happening around us. We may curl up in a fetal position. We may hide under furniture, blankets, and so on. If you are around someone experiencing a shutdown, you can help to remove them from any noisy, crowded situations, avoid asking questions that require a lot of verbal processing, don't trivialize or blame the person for the situation, and offer something that makes them comfortable (stim toy, weighted blanket, iPad, etc.).

If someone who is experiencing a shutdown asks you to leave, do it. Try to avoid asking "what's wrong?" or any variation thereof. It is not easy to describe things while having a shutdown. Please remember, every autistic person is different. Listen and be receptive to their needs. Asking simple "Yes" or "No" questions can be very helpful.

Shutdowns, and an unprepared medical system

I experienced the events of my first catastrophic shutdown while living and working in Germany. Early-1990s German socialized medicine did not appreciate or accommodate foreigners who needed significant medical care. The authorities invited me to leave the country and to not return. It was the best thing for me as I needed help, and that help wasn't available in Germany's rural south.

Back in the US, and in and out of the hospital, prior to DSM-IV and a proper diagnosis, I was still wandering. I bought a pile of Volkswagen parts that a friend and I put together into a camping Combi. I had the platform for some amazing wandering and foraging. Away I went.

A series of low-paying and rather menial jobs earned me just enough to explore. I wasn't interested in riches; I am, after all, a forager. I had mobile shelter – my Combi. I had all that I needed.

The next phase of my wandering life ties into the memory of my Uncle Sandy and occurred around the time my brain was starting to understand the verbal world. I was an emerging language learner when I was invited into employment with the city of Los Angeles to a position very much like that of my venerable relative. First, as a type of communication electrician working independently in support of various operations, I was paid handsomely to work in and around the city. Then, after 9/11, when technology and the laws were changing rapidly, I was asked to figure out an aspect of digital/multimedia evidence and became one of the founders of the digital/multimedia forensic sciences. Along the way, I penned a book, co-authored another, and wrote dozens of research papers and thousands of articles.

Being at the forefront of the discipline, and largely creating the curriculum on how to do what I was doing, I was offered opportunities to travel the world to teach those who wanted training in this new science. Away I went. As time progressed, I was invited into private forensic science casework, further enhancing my ability to explore.

I've been to most US states. I've been to Canada. I've assisted in cases from around the globe. I've even worked in South Africa – and was privileged to explore the bush surrounding its capital city.

With all of this in mind, this introduction is akin to the present me leaving this set of notes for the future me, reconciling the past me, and depositing an artifact for parents of autistic children and researchers trying to understand this pathological desire: that we solitary foragers often like to wander off.

Some who know me may read this and recall the events I've briefly outlined entirely differently. That's fine. This retelling is a reframing, inserting new information as to **why**… trying to better understand the **what**. I've always been a solitary forager.

I've just gotten better at hiding it, or better able to engage with it safely, as I've gotten older.

Glasser's Choice Theory (see the note at the end of the chapter), the theory that we are always seeking to satisfy one or more of five basic human needs, explains why we autistics choose to do what we do better than any other theoretical construct. Many of us need to wander, to explore. As Reser notes, it's biological – written into our genetic heritage. We seemingly ignore safety needs (there goes Maslow). We seemingly care not for esteem and affection. We care so deeply about exploring (or roaming) the world in the peace of solitude. Perhaps this is related to our sensory issues – the often-overwhelming noise that bombards us in crowded places.

It's important to note here that every autistic person is different in their foraging aspects. For example, some sensory seekers ignore safety needs and taste or eat things that are dangerous. On the other hand, some sensory avoiders wouldn't consider leaving their houses and must be convinced to venture out. Again, autism is a spectrum. But we can use Choice Theory and the Solitary Forager Hypothesis to help make sense of what an autistic person is doing at a given point, for example, what need(s) are they attempting to satisfy?

So why these rather personal notes? Throughout the book, I will use my rather eclectic mix of experiences to illustrate what it is to be autistic, especially as place changes. These notes are here as a preview, as a way for you, the reader, to get to know me better so that we can have a long conversation about autism. They also serve as "the mass," or the object of study. After all, by way of example, it's next to impossible to learn to fix a modern automobile from a textbook alone. You'll need to be in front of the car, hands-on. Providing my own experiences as a template can serve to give you something tangible with which to work and process the information provided in this text.

With these things in mind, the relationship between place, neurotype, and identity is quite important. In the modern Western world, one receives a diagnosis of autism based upon how one is "impacted by autism" within a certain context or place (e.g., work or school). Indeed, the diagnostic criteria, discussed later in this book, relate specifically to place. You will find, or you may already know, that within the DSM or the ICD, there is no place for autism as an identity. This fact frames the title of this book as well as its driving question. There are obvious implications to this point of view that will be explored later.

Autism and place

In this book, we're going to investigate something that may be new to you. So few of us have the privilege of wandering about the world and living authentically in a variety of spaces. Many of us can explore but need extensive supports. Indeed, in each of the contexts in which I have lived or worked, my autistic strengths and weaknesses have affected me differently. What I didn't know during the period in which I lacked knowledge of how my system works, back before my awareness that I am autistic and what that means, is how much the many aspects of place impact my experience of it.

I can drive a car now, though it terrifies me. I prefer to drive alone with the music amplified to a borderline unsafe volume. I love the feeling of music. I can blast my favorite mix of liquid drum and bass and drive for hours. Yet, I can only last a few hours at a concert before the energy of the place is so overwhelming that I begin to melt down. I have hearing protection (EarPro) that can help when I'm in required situations like my school's graduation, held in a multipurpose room with horrible acoustics. But EarPro gets in the way of experiencing the full dynamic range of music. Thus, place impacts my enjoyment of my favorite music.

As we move through this book, you will see just how well social geography can help us in the framing of discussions of the autistic experience.

The study of autism

I want to begin with a simple exercise and ask what should be a simple question: why study autism? To answer this question, you may scan your favorite dictionary and look up the word "study." There, you will likely find that to "study" is to apply the mind to or to read and examine for the purpose of learning and understanding. What about autism? What definition did you find? Likely, you found that autism or Autism Spectrum Disorder is a neurodevelopmental condition or disorder of variable severity with lifelong effects that can be recognized from early childhood by various subjective tests. The literature notes that it is chiefly characterized by difficulties with social interaction and communication and by restricted or repetitive patterns of thought and behavior (Campisi et al., 2018; Lord et al., 2018, 2020).

These definitions of autism are reductive. They're dehumanizing. They're devoid of context. They are written by the "victor" over the "vanquished." These definitions are not generally informed by autistic people. They omit identity entirely.

Because of this, we will work together to create a more comprehensive, ethical, and equitable picture of what autism is. To accomplish our task, we may have to dive deep into some uncomfortable spaces. This is normal when examining marginalized communities. Autistics of my generation were not treated well. First- and second-generation therapies were often quite abusive. Many were left with complex PTSD, myself included. But therapies have come a long way. The latest methods found in vocational and occupational rehabilitation are quite helpful. Indeed, were it not for the help of such specialists, the task of writing this book would not have been possible for me.

Our work will follow a spiraling trajectory. As we find new information, it may inform changes to previously held assumptions. We'll continually modify our premises. We may get to the end of our work having a completely new idea of what the autistic experience and identity looks like. This may cause problems in our personal lives and professional careers. I remember hearing someone say something profound on this topic, the essence of which ultimately changed one's life. They said, paraphrasing the great Rev. Dr Martin Luther King, "the truth shall set you free. But first, it will make you angry." What will you do with this truth?

Course outline

Here's how we will work our way through the course.

- **What is autism?** Working from the premise that the autistic system is the result of approximately 50,000 years of natural selection, we posit that the autistic system works as designed, and then unpack the design. The implications of this design-centric approach are explored with human geography and place identity in mind.

- **When is autism?** We will explore the human genetic record to attempt to pin down a date when autism first appeared on Earth. Once determined, we work forward in time to explore the many times and places in which autism was instrumental in the preservation of humanity.

- **Where is autism?** Understanding that autism is present in all cultures, and across the gender spectrum, we explore human geography and place identity from the standpoint of the autistic experience of place. We will find that some places are more hostile to autistic systems, and some are more accommodating.

- **Who is autistic?** Given the changing criteria for diagnosing autism in the Western world, we will explore how place influences access to this vital piece of the autistic identity. We will then move beyond the West to discover how people of other cultures identify and include (or not) the autistic people who inhabit their spaces.

- **Why autism?** Here, an exploration of diagnosis and self-diagnosis is presented. We will investigate why someone may freely choose to be a part of a community that is often on the margins of society. We will also explore the benefits and pitfalls of self-diagnosis, and why it is becoming more popular. All the while, we will consider how place influences access to diagnosis and diagnostic prevalence.

- **Summary.** Here, we hope to achieve a cohesive and humane view of autism. We finish with a **charge** – what to do with this new information.

Why study autism in this way?

The textbooks of my childhood all operated in the same way. An authority informed the reader as to the way things are. Students read the books and teachers guided their assimilation into the dominant culture. Thinking back on an earlier statement made in this introduction, if you've met one autistic person, you've met one autistic person... once. There is no way, even with more than 50 years of lived experience, that one person could hope to summarize autism authentically. Likewise, there's no way that an honest attempt at a book on autism could be crafted that focuses on one geographic area or culture. How autistic students are treated in Los Angeles, where I teach, is different than how they're treated in Idaho and Iowa, or India. Thus, we will lay out a framework and guiding questions that will help you build a view of autism that is valid for your local context while helping you understand the autistic identity within a variety of contexts.

- If you are a teacher, when you gain proficiency with this way of working, you will be able to not only empathize with autistic students but be able to understand what is necessary when creating differentiated lessons. To truly embrace Universal Design, one must know the target audience and target student. You will use the knowledge and wisdom gained through this learning process to inform your lesson planning, allowing you to create rich and engaging learning experiences.
- If you are a relative or friend of an autistic person, when you gain proficiency with this way of working, you will be able to understand your loved one at a level not previously possible. After all, we are creating what can amount to an owner's

guide to the autistic system during the learning that we will do together. This information can help you interpret autistic behaviors, actions, or intentions through an autistic lens.

- If you are autistic, you may be just beginning in your dive into what it means to be autistic. If you're non-verbal, like me, you may find the work we do here helpful in building those scripts necessary to have conversations about what you are feeling, and why. You may find the information helpful in informing your care team in effective ways of supporting you – like the proper language to use when requesting accommodations from your college.

Preparing to study

Now let's set up your notebook for the way in which we will operate throughout this exploration.

The beginning of each chapter includes a quick summary of what we will work on. Use this information to anchor your work. This summary supports the Student Learning Objective (SLO). The SLO is the thing you'll be able to do or understand once you have completed the work in the chapter. In writing the objectives for this text, I've chosen objectives at the "create" level of Bloom's Taxonomy. Benjamin Bloom and his collaborators published a framework for categorizing educational goals called the Taxonomy of Educational Objectives in 1956. The "create" level is the highest level, where one produces new or original work (Armstrong, 2022). As such, we want to put together elements and parts to form a cohesive whole, contributing to an ever-evolving look at autism and the autistic identity. If you prefer to write or type your notes, this information can be transcribed at the beginning of each chapter's notes.

Next, you may have noticed that I included a note that some key terms, optional reading selections, and references are located at the end of the chapter. Each chapter has these valuable resources. I don't assume that you will know the more technical or advanced concepts within our discussion space. Knowing full well the frustration and anxiety that can occur when encountering a new term that lacks context or definition, I build these terms and concepts into the learner experience. You may choose to transfer these to your notes. I strongly suggest that you do. The act of "writing" is so powerful in moving information from the short-term memory spaces of our brain to the long-term spaces where meaning is made and operationalized.

As we work through the chapter, you will be presented with discussion questions and inquiry activities. These should be placed in your notes in whatever way you feel is appropriate. Some like detailed notes. Others like skeletons meant to trigger memory recall. There is no one way to take notes. Depending upon how you are using this text, and in what context, you may find that typing out your notes and being as comprehensive as possible will assist you in creating and preparing professional development learning experiences of your own. Again, it's up to you how you choose to engage with the work outside of any specific guidance your local instructor, if any, may provide.

Here are three things you need to know about the work in which we will engage.

1. **Science evolves.** A scientific concept, trusted as fact in Victorian England, probably hasn't survived as fact today. For example, scientists James Glaisher and Henry Tracey Coxwell believed that they could take their hot air balloon

into space. Sir John Lubbock, Vice Chancellor of London University, spent hundreds of research hours trying to teach his dog to read. Neither worked. Science evolves, and so should we.

2. **Identity is personal.** A person's identity is the concept they develop about themself that evolves over the course of their life. It is how they define themself, not how they are defied by some external entity. As an example, a person may identify as autistic. This is how I choose to identify. Others may choose to identify as a person with autism. Both are valid when each is freely chosen by the holder of the identity. One becomes invalid when it's attributed to someone without their consent.

3. **Autism is the English word for an experience and an identity.** Autism is called "takiwātanga," meaning "his or her own time and space," by New Zealand's Māori (Opai, 2017). In Mandarin, the word autism (自閉症) is made from the pictograms for "one's self" (自), "to close or obstruct" (verb) (閉), and "disease" (症). Thus, when researching autism in various local contexts, it is important to know how autism is referred to locally. It is also important to understand the context in which the word was brought into each language. In the case of Māori, great care was made to choose a word that did not have a negative connotation. In Mandarin, however, its name has clear clinical connotations.

During our studies

As we work through this book, you will be asked to do research. Researching is not something that comes naturally to people. Whenever possible, I will include the appropriate search criteria and suggest locations in which the most helpful information can be found. Depending on where you live and how you are engaging with this text, you may not have access to the search engine or data set suggested. Understanding this, I'll also suggest possible workarounds or alternate locations.

Follow along as I illustrate how this might look.

- Browse to scholar.google.com. Enter **"autism identity"** into the search field and either press the magnifying glass on the page or press the enter key on your keyboard. Make a note of the titles of the top three results. Click on your browser's back button. Enter **"autism"** and **"identity"** into the search field and either press the magnifying glass on the page or press the enter key on your keyboard. Here, we separate autism and identity as unique search terms by putting quotes around them and including the word "and" as an operator. Notice the titles of the top three results. Are they different? It is likely they're quite different. During our work, you will gain expertise in the science of searches.

- Choose one of the results from your last search. If you chose one of the top listings, it is likely that the data that you are after is behind a paywall. The big journal publishing companies often charge upwards of US$50 for a journal article. If you lack institutional access to the journal, research can become quite expensive. There are two ways around it. The first is PubMed, a free search engine hosted in the US by its National Library of Medicine. As much of the research around autism will be found in medical journals, searching PubMed (as opposed to Google Scholar) will give you access to more information and abstracts for free. The second is to make a note of the paper's author(s). Many are easy to find through their university. Send them a note and ask if they will send you a copy of the paper you would like to use. Take it from me, a PhD holder, I am always happy to help other researchers. I frequently share copies of my research with those honestly working to make the world a better place for us autistics.

Check for understanding

How are you doing? Were there any words or terms that you didn't understand? Pause a beat. Then, after a few seconds, write them down in your notes. If you are part of the neurodivergent community, what I am about to recommend will come naturally. Launch your favorite browser and look up those words or terms.

- What results do you find? Include them in your notes. They may prove useful later.
- How do you feel about what you found? Was it easy? Did you have to try multiple times to get what you were looking for? What does this effort suggest about the word you are looking for?

Did anything in this introduction trigger an emotional response in you? If so, sit with it. Invite it into the theater of your mind, into your imagination. Ask it what it hopes to accomplish. See where your mind goes. You may find yourself not quite understanding where your mind goes. The subconscious does not obey physical reality's rules. It may take some practice to work effectively in the theater of the mind. But it is a powerful tool. You may choose to skip ahead briefly to Chapter 5 where this is explored in further depth.

Some things that might trip you up

There are some common issues that researchers of autism come upon which can have profound implications if not recognized and dealt with early on. Engaging with them may also lead to personal consequences. Thus, a bit of a trigger warning is necessary. Some uncomfortable conversations are about to happen.

- Many autistic people do not have access to the internet. When I say this, I am framing the statement in a worldwide context. Thus, the autistic community cannot be polled accurately on Twitter. Much of what constitutes the "autistic community" online consists of privileged people from what we consider Western cultures. Thus, one of the ways in which we will accomplish our learning goals is to help build that body of knowledge and resources that can assist you in building an inclusive local community right where you live.

- Being autistic is often not always fun. Being disabled never is. There have been plenty of times where I wished that I was neurotypical. Many autistic people privately admit this. Some, like me, will publicly acknowledge just how many times they've wanted to be "like everyone else." Author Elizabeth Moon, in her best-selling book *The Speed of Dark*, explores a scenario whereby autism has been cured by genetic alteration. The main character is of a generation of autistics that wasn't genetically altered before birth. He's given an opportunity to receive that treatment, thus "curing" him. I won't spoil the ending. But the story raises some important issues. In your work, you will likely encounter neurotypical parents of neurodivergent children. Their experiences are an important part of the discussion on what it means to be autistic. They have valuable information on how place impacts the autistic identity. Thus, you will want to get to know them and their child/children. Yet, many in the so-called "actually autistic community" dismiss these "Autism Moms" as not having a place in the conversation. In places like Facebook, Instagram, and Twitter, the interaction between these two camps can get quite vicious, with the autistic side often being the aggressors.

We can work through these issues if we are open to honest conversations. When you discover that in some societies, an autism diagnosis is a terrible thing that no family wants for their child, how will it inform your discussions with a local family about advocating for a diagnosis for their child? How did the other society's framing of the issues, why they think autism is a bad thing, inform your local conversations?

We can see this at work in a seemingly horrific example from the COVID-19 pandemic and the response of the National Health Service (NHS) in the United Kingdom. There, at the peak of the pandemic, where there was a severe shortage of resources, some autistic people were encouraged to have a Do Not Resuscitate health directive by their local clinic (BBC, 2020). The likely cause of the directives lies in the belief that autistic (disabled) lives weren't as essential, and thus should be sacrificed so that the more vital could be saved. The conversation in the autistic community in the UK wondered what might happen if an autistic person was admitted to hospital without a directive. Would the NHS see the diagnosis in the system and refuse to provide more than basic care? While there are no reports that autistics were refused services, this scenario was real. These discussions did happen.

In situations where health care must be rationed, it's often the disabled who suffer the most.

End of chapter activity

Now it's your turn. With what you've learned, and with what you already know, explore the evolution of your own intersectional identities as your place/context has changed over time. Create a few paragraphs that summarize this evolution. Here are some ideas to consider as you engage with the exercise.

- Consider the name you were given at birth. Do you still use that name? If not, what name do you use, why do you use it, and when did the change take place? As a way of illustrating a response, I prefer to use the diminutive of my middle name. I've never used my first name in any way except formally. My family knows me by a nickname that very few know of or use.

- Consider using one of the many online intersectionality calculators. After interacting with one, what do you think of the experience? What do you think of the results? Do they seem oversimplified or accurate?

- Consider where you live now. Are you within 20 miles of where you were born? How often have you moved (e.g., living situations, neighborhoods, cities, and countries), if at all? Are there places where you felt you could be more of yourself than others? How did that make you feel? If you no longer live in a place where you didn't feel comfortable, did you move because of that fact?

These certainly aren't the only elements of identity that you can explore. They're placed here to get the conversation started.

Please feel free to take your exploration of place and identity where it feels most appropriate.

Summary

In this introductory chapter, I introduced myself and offered samples of my unique lived experience of being a non-verbal autistic person across various contexts. We were introduced to the concept of intersectionality and how identity can be fluid as place and time change. The discussions and reflections that likely took place around the information presented herein should have helped you to be able to synthesize, albeit simply, what autism can look like in your local context as well as in other places.

With the introduction complete, we move on to dive deeper into what autism is, what it isn't, and how the definitions and diagnostic criteria we have now evolved and continue to evolve.

Key vocabulary and terms

- **DSM.** The Diagnostic and Statistical Manual of Mental Disorders (DSM) is a publication by the American Psychiatric Association (APA). Its current version is DSM-5-TR.

- **Flow state.** Often misinterpreted as "low functioning" in autism, flow states are a sense of fluidity between one's body and mind, where one is totally absorbed by and deeply focused on something, beyond the point of distraction. Here, the perception of time is irrelevant. The senses are heightened. The person in a flow state is at one with the task at hand, with action and awareness synchronizing to create effortless and unbounding energy. Some people would describe this feeling as being "in the zone." Associated with monotropism in the scientific literature.

- **Glasser's Choice Theory.** Dr William Glasser's Choice Theory states that all human behavior is driven by the desire to satisfy five basic human needs:

  o the need to be loved and accepted;

  o the need to be powerful;

  o the need to be free;

  o the need to have fun; and

  o the need to survive.

- **Human geography (aka anthropogeography).** A branch of geography that examines people and their relationships with communities, cultures, and economies, as well as interactions with their environment by studying their relations with and across locations.

- **ICD.** The World Health Organization's International Statistical Classification of Diseases and Related Health Problems (ICD) is the global standard for diagnostic health information. It is currently in its 11th revision.

- **Info-dump (info-dumping).** Common among autistic people, info-dumping is the practice of giving intricately detailed and perhaps overly long summaries of their special interest. Info-dumping is also known as "speaking in paragraphs."

- **Inspiration porn.** A term created by the late disability activist Stella Young, it refers to the objectification of people with disabilities in the media, which serves the purpose of making people without disabilities feel good. There are several types of inspiration porn. One occurs when a disabled person receives praise for participating in a "normal" activity or event.

Another type occurs when a disabled person "overcomes" their disability to take part in a specific activity. Still another type occurs when a disabled person receives assistance from a non-disabled person and then the non-disabled person is glorified for their "service to humanity."

- **Intersectionality.** A framework in sociology that outlines the processes through which multiple identities intersect or overlap, affecting the lives of individuals and/or groups.

- **Neurodivergent.** Someone who differs in mental or neurological function from what is considered typical or normal. There are lots of ways to be neurodivergent: OCD, ADHD, autistic, dyslexic, and so on. Someone who is not neurotypical may be considered neurodivergent.

- **Neurodiverse.** A group of people who differ in mental or neurological function from what is considered typical or normal. The group should include different neurodivergent identities to be considered neurodiverse. For an individual to be considered neurodiverse, they should have multiple co-occurring neurological-based diagnoses.

- **Neurotypical.** Someone who does not display autistic or other neurologically atypical patterns of thought or behavior.

- **Social geography.** A branch of human geography that examines the relationships between society and space or place.

- **Solitary forager.** A term taken from Jared Reser's 2011 paper, "Conceptualizing the autism spectrum in terms of natural selection and behavioral ecology: The solitary forager hypothesis," found in *Evolutionary Psychology*, 9(2), pp. 207–238. His paper reviewed etiological and comparative evidence supporting the hypothesis that some heritable genes associated with what we now call the autism spectrum were naturally selected and represent the adaptive benefits of being cognitively suited for solitary foraging.

- **The Quality World.** Part of Glasser's Choice Theory, one's Quality World is one's idea or mental picture of their perfect life. Unique to the individual, one's Quality World is a place in their mind where they store mental images of what they find important. Glasser believed that these pictures in a person's Quality World make them feel good, meeting at least one of the five basic needs. An important note, these pictures need not align with society's standards or values.

Building background knowledge

The following titles are not required reading but will serve those who study this topic by providing valuable context and background knowledge.

Glasser, W. (1998). *Choice Theory: A New Psychology of Personal Freedom*. New York: Harper Perennial.

Reser, J. (2011). Conceptualizing the autism spectrum in terms of natural selection and behavioral ecology: The solitary forager hypothesis. *Evolutionary Psychology: An International Journal of Evolutionary Approaches to Psychology and Behavior*, 9(2), pp. 207–238.

2
What is autism?

Learning objective

Students will be able to describe autism as both a set of traits and as an identity using place identity to guide their work.

Activity

Students research and report on how autism is presented in academic literature. From where do most of the studies originate? Students explore the implications of their answers. Additionally, the implications of person-first/identity-first language are explored.

Introduction

In the previous chapter, I shared that I am a multi-sport athlete. I'll use that bit of information here to build a shared understanding of an important concept that we'll need to move forward in our discussion of autism. Before I begin, you're likely wondering, what does the author's athletic history have to do with autism? The answer is simple. Athletes, however skilled, will get injured and must seek medical care. You'll see in a moment what this has to do with autism.

Years ago, I was playing basketball in a competitive league. The opposing team was full of amazingly talented players, and I was often struggling to keep up with my counterpart on defense. One missed shot by my teammate led to a fast break and I was trailing behind the man with the ball. As he went to lay the ball up, I rushed in from behind to block the shot. My body's trajectory, speed, and the motion of my arm were in perfect position to make the block. Unfortunately, my hand and wrist were out of position. My thumb struck the ball, pinning it violently to the backboard. The force of that event concentrated in my wrist, completely and painfully rearranging the small bones and connective tissue.

I arrived at hospital writhing in pain. I told the intake nurse what had happened. I extended my arm so he could see the damage for himself. The doctor ordered diagnostic exams. The X-ray technician winced at the sight of my wrist, as shown in the films. I was given a cast and scheduled for surgery. Guided by the diagnostic information, the surgeon expertly rearranged my wrist, restoring it to a function of about 80 percent of normal. Later, physical therapy helped get me back to almost 100 percent.

Unbeknownst to me at the time, there was a dizzying array of forms that accompanied all these events at the hospital. Each step had its medical code. Each pill, pin, device, and procedure has its code in order that records are properly kept, and everyone gets paid. Nosography provides the descriptions and nosology provides the classifications. For my disfigured wrist, the diagnostic criteria, as well as the pathway to a restoration to a proper functioning joint, were clear. In the Western medical system, a similarly trained and equipped set of professionals could examine my wrist, come to a diagnosis and treatment plan, and provide me with the same outcome. Such is the standardization in Western physical medicine.

With my wrist, the straightforward identification procedure leads to the generation of a billing code. For a displaced fracture of the middle third of the navicular bone of an unspecified wrist, the initial encounter for a closed fracture, S62.023A, is the billable/specific ICD-10-CM code that can be used to indicate a diagnosis for reimbursement purposes. This magic code is necessary and guides the treatment. In the hospital billing system, there are procedures and expendables connected with having such a diagnosis that the system accepts and will pay for. It will pay for X-rays, splints, and physical therapy for the wrist. It won't pay for mammograms, eyeglasses, or alcohol rehabilitation as none of those things are related to the initial billing event – the fractured wrist.

Having the correct diagnosis, and the correct billing code, makes all the difference in the world when seeking health care. When we look at an autism diagnosis, we must understand that there isn't an X-ray, blood test, or MRI scan that can indicate to a doctor that one is autistic. How we each arrive at our autism diagnosis is rather unique to each of us and is heavily dependent on the place in which we seek it (Wen et al., 2022). For those without a diagnosis, but a self-identification, access to supports and accommodations that are vital to health and happiness is often elusive (Davies et al., 2022).

The diagnosis of autism spectrum disorder

There were no diagnostic codes for autism when I was a child. Autistic people of my generation, and older, were "weird," "shy," "quiet," "odd," and sometimes quite "clumsy." I certainly was all those things. Our parents would often remark that our traits would make it difficult for us to find work, that we should work on our social graces, and our peculiarities often embarrassed them in public (Fang et al., 2022). Parents being parents, they worried about us. Being a parent of an autistic child can be quite stressful (Mumtaz, Fatima, and Saqulain, 2022). They didn't always have a loving way of showing it, but they did want the best for us then as modern parents do now (Marriott et al., 2022). My having a war veteran as a parent brought the concept that the military might straighten me out and make me a fit member of society.

Growing up as I did in the US working class, the military is always present as an option of employment leading to a trade or a skill. Not being literate, and not really liking the academic aspects of school, I thought to myself as I grew up that I would join the US Navy and be an aircraft engine mechanic. I thought that I could leverage my systematizing mind to facilitate a career with an organization that itself wanders the world. In my teen years, the local recruiter made assurances about my choice of vocation as I made my plans to enter military service. Being satisfied that my future direction would be secure, I signed up for military service. The induction process began. Regardless of the branch, the first stop in the induction process is always the entrance physical.

I went through all the indignities associated with physical exams done in a stadium setting and ended up in the hearing test area. I was told to put the headset on and when I heard the tones to press the button on the remote that they had handed me, I heard tones. I pressed the button. I thought everything was going well throughout the test. But, at its conclusion, the Marine who was running the test told me angrily to "stop f-ing around."

He demanded I retake the test. I did. Same test. Same results. Angrier Marine. "Listen, jagoff," he said. "You've only got one more chance to get this right. No more f-ing around." Same test. Same results. Even angrier Marine. "Congratulations, sh-thead," he said. "You failed." With a failure of the hearing test, I was disqualified from service.

I had no idea why I failed the test. But its failure meant that I would have to sort out a different future. At 6'5" and 265 lbs., I easily settled on college football.

Moving forward a decade or so, I entered police service in early 2001. Part of that process was a vision and hearing screening. I had the same issues in the hearing test in 2001 as I did in 1986. But this time, the audio technician was entirely more helpful than the foul-mouthed Marine. She said that she didn't think I had "hearing loss," but rather a hearing "delay." Because I was able to hear speech, and have a conversation with her, she would note the "delay," but not disqualify me from service due to "hearing loss." She recommended I see an audiologist for a proper diagnosis.

Getting the job, a rather well-paying job at that, meant having access to health care through my new employer. With that access, I could investigate this hearing delay. Appointments were made and screenings performed. The various audiologists were puzzled by the results. The structures of my ear were perfectly healthy. There was a delay or confusion happening. They figured that it was "all in my head." They recommended that I see someone in behavioral health to see if the condition was somehow psychological.

Within behavioral health, I was taken through a variety of screening questionnaires. I saw a team of specialists. At the end of it all, a psychiatrist sat me down to give me the answers to all my questions. It was a four-hour-long conversation.

He told me that he suspected I had a condition known alternately as either Sensory Processing Disorder or Sensory Integration Disorder. That, regarding my "hearing delay," the sensations of sound were not arriving in the right place and time. These auditory signals were not being processed by my brain correctly. The problem, he noted, was that there was disagreement within the psychiatric community as to whether either of these conditions existed. Getting treatment required a billable diagnosis. Some of his colleagues outside of my medical plan, he noted, have had success with listing the condition as "other disorders of psychological development (diagnostic/billing code F88)." But my plan didn't recognize that billing code as reimbursable.

Because the team had suspected other issues at play, some of the screening tools were looking for the presence of what were then termed as pervasive developmental disorders. Given the results, he said to me, he believed that I had Asperger's Syndrome (also known as Asperger's Disorder). The ICD-10 code for the diagnosis Asperger's Syndrome was F84.5 and was a valid diagnostic/billing code in their system. He listed my diagnosis as Asperger's Syndrome with the presence of Sensory Integration Disorder. With the diagnosis, I could get help and my health plan would pay for it.

As I dove into the diagnosis, so many unanswered questions were answered. I experienced the sense of relief that many autistic people do when they receive confirmation that something is indeed different about them. Later, when DSM-IV became DSM-5, all the pervasive development disorders suddenly became autism spectrum disorder. In the billing system of my health plan, Asperger's went away – replaced by autism. Now, with the Text Revision to DSM-5, we're left wondering about what changes will happen for those of us with an ASD diagnosis. But we'll get to that question in depth later in the book. As for my new diagnostic/billing code, I was and am the proud owner of 6A02.2, Autism spectrum disorder without disorder of intellectual development and with impaired functional language.

A quick view of how the Western medical systems view autism

What I am going to present here might be new to you. It might be triggering to some. Nevertheless, any examination of autism must include multiple perspectives. In this case, we begin with how the Western medical systems view autism. There are, of course, other viewpoints and frameworks. There are Black, Brown, Indigenous communities who don't align with neoliberal, Western cultures that center individual identity labels. These cultures wonder if people should even take on a neurodivergent or neurotypical label. These labels serve no purpose in their cultures. They often recoil at the thought that one of these labels be assigned to someone by default (Khan, 2022).

As we've seen, for those in neoliberal Western cultures whose identity is focused on autism, it's hard to hear that the medical establishment believes there to be a rather standard human experience. In this view, the medical model of disability, the standard human experience is altered negatively by some external force. With autism, when seen as a pervasive developmental disorder, the normal mental development of the child is slowed. Communication is impacted. Other problems are present that need treatment. Parents are advised that intensive work will need to happen if they hope to give their disabled child a chance in life.

At this point in the discussion, it may be helpful to define who "they" are. Who comprises this system that assigns diagnoses? While psychiatrists or psychologists offer diagnoses, the two organizations who create and maintain the list of diagnostic criteria and billing codes are the American Psychiatric Association (APA) and the World Health Organization (WHO). The APA is responsible for the DSM and the WHO is responsible for the ICD. These two groups have an entirely different focus and entirely different goals. For example, DSM-III and ICD-8 were worlds apart in content and tone. Over time, the two groups have worked together such that DSM-5-TR and ICD-11 are quite harmonious (Bradley, 2013).

Yet, important distinctions remain. The ICD is produced by a body of the world's experts, while the DSM is published by an American trade group (the APA). This means that the ICD's development is a global, multidisciplinary, and multicultural process while the development of the DSM happens within a single Western country's context. Importantly, the ICD is distributed around the world at a very low cost. Its text is available free on the internet. The WHO does not depend upon it for revenue. By contrast, the DSM generates a very significant portion of the APA's annual revenue. Nevertheless, the DSM is still viewed worldwide as the diagnostic "bible." It contains information that will never be part of the ICD. Thus, it's important to understand the place and function of both systems.

The APA's DSM-5-TR provides standardized criteria to help diagnose what it terms as 299.00 Autism Spectrum Disorder. To meet the diagnostic criteria for ASD according to DSM-5-TR, a child must have persistent deficits in each of three areas of social communication and interaction (Section A: social-emotional reciprocity; non-verbal communicative behaviors used for social interaction; and developing, maintaining, and understanding relationships) plus all the types of restricted, repetitive behaviors (Section B: stereotyped or repetitive motor movements, use of objects, or speech; insistence on sameness, inflexible adherence to routines, or ritualized patterns of verbal or non-verbal behavior; highly restricted, fixated interests that are abnormal in intensity or focus; and hyper- or hypo-reactivity to sensory input or unusual interests in sensory aspects of the environment). The severity levels are in place to indicate the level of support that will be necessary to bring the child to a baseline functioning level within a typical environment (e.g., home or school). The specific criteria can be found by a quick search of the internet. The US Centers for Disease Control and Prevention's website helped inform the creation of this book (CDC, 2022).

By way of comment, the previous version of the DSM, DSM-5, noted that clinicians need only observe and record two of the four criteria in Section B. The Text Revision's "clarification" of Section B to declare that all four criteria must be observed and recorded will likely result in a reduced number of diagnoses. Additionally, the emphasis on early diagnosis, combined with the "clarification," will inevitably lead to fewer adults receiving a diagnosis. Consider that by the time an autistic person has reached adulthood, they've likely developed many coping mechanisms and communications workarounds to cope with a place that offers little/no accommodations that the system may no longer see them as impaired or disabled (Woods, 2017). As we will explore later, diagnosis is entirely place dependent.

As verbose as the DSM is in its diagnostic criteria, the ICD seems spartan. "Autism spectrum disorder is characterized by persistent deficits in the ability to initiate and to sustain reciprocal social interaction and social communication, and by a range of restricted, repetitive, and inflexible patterns of behaviour and interests" (WHO, 2022).

ICD-11 also notes that there are "several sub-types of autism spectrum disorder, depending on levels of intellectual and language development. This encompasses the whole range of ability, from individuals with high IQ and good language to those with intellectual disability and no functional language" (WHO, 2022).

The professionals who are generally authorized to diagnose ASD can be found among the ranks of developmental pediatricians, developmental-behavioral pediatricians, child psychologists, child psychiatrists, occupational therapists, or pediatric neurologists (Royal Children's Hospital Melbourne, 2022). Depending upon the laws of the countries in which they practice, these professionals must often possess an additional authorization to their license to perform such diagnostics (Therapeutic Pathways, 2021). Unfortunately for adults, the process is focused on diagnosing children as young as possible. For adults, psychologists and psychiatrists can diagnose ASD in certain situations or within some health care plans. They will likely have received additional training on ASD. Additionally, in the US and several other Western countries, a licensed and certified rehabilitation counselor can provide a diagnosis. Often, the diagnosis is a result of a collaborative effort of a team of professionals conducting interviews with relatives, friends, and classmates/colleagues.

An important point to remember is that autism has no concrete diagnostic criteria as such. At the present time, there are no medical tests (e.g., blood or imaging) that can diagnose autism. Currently, autism is diagnosed by the above-referenced clinicians who administer autism-specific behavioral evaluations. In addition to their own observations, these professionals also rely on the observations of parents or relatives, physicians, and therapists to learn as much as they can about the person in question to make a diagnosis. It's a qualitative judgment, not a quantitative analysis. It's entirely subjective and not at all objective.

Diagnostic tools

The primary tools used in the diagnosis of ASD in Western countries are as follows:

- DISCO – Diagnostic Interview for Social and Communication Disorders (Leekam et al., 2002);
- ADI-R – Autism Diagnostic Interview–Revised (Rutter, LeCouteur, and Lord, 2003, 2008);
- ADOS – Autism Diagnostic Observation Schedule (Hus and Lord, 2014); and
- 3Di – Developmental, Dimensional, and Diagnostic Interview (Skuse et al., 2004).

With those tools, the clinician(s) will make a diagnosis of ASD based on:

- the criteria from the diagnostic manuals;
- the information from the diagnostic tools; and
- their own professional judgment.

These tools can vary in price from free to almost US$20,000 to license for clinical use. They aren't the only tools available but remain the most popular. Below are some screening tools that are available online at either low or no cost to the user. Obviously, if one is using the tools to self-diagnose, their conclusions do not receive the weight and authority of a formal diagnosis from a licensed professional. Nevertheless, they are helpful when initially seeking answers to those "why do I (my loved one) feel this way" questions.

The most popular ASD screening tests:

- AQ-10 – Short Autism Quotient – 10 statements;
- AQ – Autism Quotient – 50 statements;
- EQ – Empathy Quotient – 60 statements;
- SQ – Systemizing Quotient–Revised – 75 statements;
- RAADS-R – Ritvo Autism Asperger Diagnostic Scale–Revised – 80 statements;
- The Aspie Quiz – 121 questions;
- CAT-Q – Camouflaging Autistic Traits Questionnaire – 25 statements; and
- RBQ-2A – Repetitive Behaviours Questionnaire – 20 statements.

Additional helpful screening tests:

- OAQ – Online Alexithymia Questionnaire – 37 statements;
- TAS-20 – Toronto Alexithymia Scale – 20 statements;
- TEQ – Toronto Empathy Questionnaire – 20 statements;
- EDA-QA – Extreme Demand Avoidance Questionnaire – 26 statements;
- ASRS-5 – ADHD Self-Report Scale for DSM-5 – 6 questions;
- VIA – VIA Inventory of Strengths – 96 statements;
- Big 5 – The Big Five Inventory-A – 44 statements;
- ESQ – Executive Skills Questionnaire – 36 statements; and
- VAS – Vulnerable Attachment Style Questionnaire – 22 statements.

Now what?

If you are not an autistic person, imagine taking all those tests. All those probing interview questions. All that energy. How soon would you melt down? How long would it take for you to quit, thinking it better to figure out how to go it alone rather than face such a gauntlet? Yet, this is the current situation. Many adults use the free tools to self-diagnose and prepare themselves for the more formal process, if they can afford it. For those with health coverage, the average time from initial inquiry to diagnosis is one year. For those without health coverage, the time factor is longer as fewer options exist outside of medical plan networks. Additionally, the costs of diagnosis outside of a medical plan can easily exceed US$5,000. Thus, an adult diagnosis in the Western world becomes a rare privilege. The result is that many diagnosed autistics received their diagnosis as a child. In the US, the age of diagnosis generally ranges from two to nine years old (Lord et al., 2006). Those that do not get an early medical diagnosis are often discovered in primary school. Inside such settings, the system can offer an "educational eligibility" for an Individualized Educational Plan (IEP) under the category of autism based on behaviors observed by the IEP team (Lightner, 2022). Parents can use the IEP to begin discussions with their care providers about a formal diagnosis.

How does the natural world view autism?

Having examined how Western societies view autism, from a deficits standpoint, we must now turn in a more philosophical direction. Considering that over long periods of time nature tends toward balance, and that the human wiring system that we now call autism is not new, what sort of natural balance is achieved in the world by having a small percentage of autistic individuals present? What imbalance might be created if autistic people were removed from the world? Contrasting with the medical model of disability, the neurodiversity paradigm suggests that neurological differences are a quite normal part of human history (Walker, 2022).

Reser posits, in his Solitary Forager Hypothesis, that upon separation from their parent(s), young autistic individuals may have been wired to seek a different life trajectory. He notes that such trajectories are common among mammals and even some primates, those of hunting and gathering primarily on their own. Thus, the many predispositions and traits that autistic individuals exhibit are viewed in Reser's hypothesis as adaptations that complement a solitary lifestyle.

Is it not interesting that there are multiple varieties of sharks, apes, gorillas, hawks… but there's only one way that nature has fashioned the human being? Does it not further stretch credulity that there is only one "right" way to be human? It does seem rather convenient that the "problems" began not too soon after the Industrial Revolution and the shift to a more urban and industrial world.

What if the autistic system works exactly as designed? If it's not a mistake, but a result of untold years of human evolution as the neurodiversity paradigm suggests, what purpose does the autistic neurological wiring plan serve? What is the purpose of a relatively solitary, intuitive, empathic, and highly intelligent being? Why aren't we spending more time working out answers to these questions instead of searching for cures and therapies? Why are we not just trying to fit a square peg into a round hole, but removing solid matter to transform the peg into something it was never designed to be?

Preparing for this chapter's activity

Having presented an introduction to autism as a "condition" or "state of being," we now turn our attention to the body of literature that informs the discussion. Our activity for this chapter asks us to research and report on how autism is presented in academic literature. You can create a graphic organizer to help you keep track of the main studies and trends. For example, you can create a row to keep track of the country of origin, with a column for individual countries. Or you can simply separate the row between the "West" and "non-West." If you limit your inquiry to the top 100 results in your search, you will find that each country is looking at autism from largely the same angle. You may choose to record the purposes of the studies in your organizer. Or you may save time and skip recording that information once you determine that the purpose of most of the top studies is to find a way to make the autistic person more desirable to some industry or other (e.g., manufacturing or education).

Indeed, place does have much to do with the focus of the studies, or even if studies are needed at all. Highly industrialized countries like the US, Canada, Australia, and the UK must sort out what should be done with that portion of their population that requires specialized care to fit in and be productive. My experience with the US military is an example where the system sees no way to accommodate my system or no use for what talents I do have. In contrast to this view, the modern state of Israel finds a way to include autistics in their military ranks. The Israel Defense Force's Ro'im Rachok program (Ono Academic College, 2022), or "viewing beyond the horizons," examines strengths and weaknesses of recruits considering its needs. Each individual recruit is evaluated to see where they might best fit in. The IDF's Unit 9900, for example, requires soldiers to have strong powers of concentration, along with strong spatial intelligence and visual perception, to decipher what they see in spatial imagery. Israeli researchers have demonstrated that the visual perception of autistic people is often different than that of neurotypicals. They have found that autistic individuals often excel at examining complex image analysis tasks objectively, focusing only on the raw data and the purpose of the analysis, without presuppositional or other such biases.

Thus, as you prepare to complete the activity, think in terms of your own context as well as more globally. Where does it seem that autistics tend to do well? Where do they suffer most? What do the answers to these questions have to say about autism and place? Does autism have a place in this world?

Important considerations

Here are some things you need to know when reviewing research around autism. Add the following data points to your graphic organizer where it makes sense to do so.

1. Very little research around autism is currently conducted by autistic people. When evaluating research, you will often find that autistic researchers self-identify in the author biography portion of the paper. Thus, you may choose to add a row to capture this data.

2. Of the institutions that fund research, very few have autistic people in positions of authority. This might take a bit of digging to find. However, groups whose primary focus is autism support usually feature the identities of their board members in their biographies. Many of these support organizations were started by the parents of autistic people hoping to eventually cure their autistic loved one. Thus, their study themes may skew in a particular direction. Nevertheless, it is an important datapoint given the power of lived experience and advocacy.

3. In the search results, pay attention to the "Cited By" number. You may choose to set up a row to capture this data. To illustrate the importance of this data, consider that Google Scholar notes that Simon Baron-Cohen's 1999 book, *Mindblindness: An Essay on Autism and Theory of Mind*, has

been cited over 10,000 times in papers about autism. Yet, Gernsbacher and Yergeau's 2019 "Empirical failures of the claim that autistic people lack a theory of mind," a paper that thoroughly rubbishes Baron-Cohen's work, has been cited in a mere 73 papers as of the writing of this book. There are myriad reasons why the problematic ideas of Baron-Cohen are pervasive, while critiques illustrating the lack of support and reproducibility of his work generate silence.

4.   Remember, in the medical model, autism is treated as a medical disorder. This model has been criticized by the neurodivergent community for looking in a negative direction, for example, on what a person cannot do instead of what they can do. You may seek to discover if the research you are examining uses the medical model in its examination and discussion of autism. Alternatively, the paper may follow the social model. In the social model, autism is simply a different way of being that often results in an autistic person being excluded from some aspects of society because of behaving differently from the expected norms. Very few use the Power Threat Meaning Framework to guide their inquiry. Those that do offer a rather refreshing view on the subject. You may choose to set up a row to capture this data, with columns for each of the models you may find in use.

5.   Finally, consider how autism is described in the piece. Do the researchers use identity-first or person-first language (Callahan, 2018)? One can easily argue for the significance of how one uses language in research, as well as potential consequences for the community under study. Does the language used seem to empower or belittle the studied group? Many autistic people believe that person-first

language is stigmatizing and dehumanizing; that it robs them of agency. Others prefer person-first language, often noting that their disability does not define them. Still, in many studies, the language is defined by the style guide of the publication. You may choose to set up a row to capture this data, with columns for each of the styles you may find in use as well as if the choice was the author's or the publication's (if that information is available).

What does this look like in practice?

Let us consider the following paper from Botha et al. (2021), "Does language matter?" The authors do not self-identify as autistic. They do, however, invite you to connect with them via their website and social media accounts. A look there shows them to be quite involved in autism research with a decided equity lens. The paper was published in the *Journal of Autism and Developmental Disorders*. The journal lists their editors and editorial board members. There is no specific statement as to any autistic identity of any of the listed members. It's a recent paper, only having been published in 2021. Thus, there aren't that many other articles that have cited it. Although not explicitly stated, the language used is consistent with those who employ the social model of disability. Finally, their work uses identity-first language.

In evaluating the paper on how it frames autism and the autistic experience, it can serve to inform discussions of the conceptualizing of autism. Indeed, the authors note how the system "sees" autism is informed by the language it uses. They contrast this view with how we autistics envision autism as both neurotype and identity that must necessarily be transferred into the verbal space in the form of words to form our descriptions. Those words must convey the sum of our lived experience and the totality of our beliefs. Are we autistic? Do we identify with our neurotype? If so, they note that we will likely choose identity-first language. It's this sort of deep-diving philosophical treatment that makes this paper a valuable addition to our body of knowledge on autism. After my review, I would thus include it in my graphic organizer.

Let's debrief what you saw

I used Google Scholar to find articles on the use of language when describing autism in the research literature, and found the above-mentioned article. I had my graphic organizer by my side as I read it, collecting data to determine if this paper was worth adding to my collection of research on the topic. I found much of what I was looking for within the paper itself. Other information, like the primary author's pronouns, for example, I found by clicking through on links at the bottom of the paper. There, I found the author's LinkedIn page and website. From there, I found information about the primary author in my attempt to determine if this paper was a one-off or if the author is actively working in this area. I found the latter to be true.

Here's where you might get tripped up

The authors engaged in a short discussion over the issue of verbal vs. speaking. If you are not familiar with the issue, you might conflate non-verbal with non-speaking, not knowing that they are two different things. Thus, we will have to do a bit of side research on the issue to discover what is being said here and, more importantly, if we agree with the premise.

At issue is communication. Communication has many different, often conflicting, meanings. It can mean the imparting or exchanging of information. It can be a means of sending or receiving information. These can be combined to form a more complex definition, the act of conveying an intended meaning to another entity using mutually understood signs and semiotic (relating to signs and symbols) rules. It's this combined definition where the problems begin between neurotypicals and autistic people – the mutual and agreed-upon understanding of signs/symbols.

You see, if you are neurotypical, you and I (the non-verbal autistic person) likely don't "speak" the same language. My typing this information, your reading this page, is a form of communication. But, because you can't "speak" my language, I must use your signs and symbols to communicate with you. This verbal/vocal form of communication wasn't always possible for me as I didn't start life knowing your "language." I had to learn. That process took a lot of time.

Remember that medical science views autism partly as a communication disorder. Based upon a growing body of research, much of the autistic population is "non-verbal" (Gernsbacher, Morson, and Grace, 2016). What that means is complex but boils down to the fact that some don't think and process in "words" but in multi-dimensional semiotics (Prizant, 1983). Imagine that what you and I consider to be the "verbal" world is like a 50 cl shot glass. How some autistics think, our multi-dimensional semiotics, is like a 150 l barrel. When a "non-verbal" person is asked a question, the final answer will occupy the entirety of a specific 150 l space. To get to the final answer, other potentially related 150 l barrels of prior knowledge and related information are assembled and the probability of the appropriate barrel, or the correct response, is calculated. Usually, it's found that a single barrel's contents aren't the appropriate choice, and thus the contents of multiple 150 l barrels are sorted and then combined appropriately. Some information is lost in the process (spills), requiring a reassembly. Then, the attempt is made to answer – effectively attempting to empty 150 l into a 50 cl shot glass without spilling a drop. It doesn't work very well.

Now imagine physically manipulating full barrels of beer. How exhausting would it be to move multiple barrels around in a short amount of time? So it is to us with vocal conversation. Making the attempt at "verbal" communication requires a lot of energy. It takes a lot of focus. It's physically exhausting. As a personal example, it's why I generally take a week to recover after teaching a 40-hour technical training session – I'm quite literally drained.

Back to the issue of "verbal" vs. "vocal." "Verbal" is not necessarily "vocal." Words can be spoken. Words can also be written. On average, autistic people are better at the written than the vocal. We can take our time. We can assemble our thoughts. Thanks to modern word processing, we can revise and edit in a non-linear fashion that isn't necessarily possible with a pen/paper or a typewriter.

Many parents seek help for their non-vocal autistic children (Kim, 2022). Speech delay is a common thing for autistics. There may be many reasons the child is not vocalizing as the parents expect. They may have a non-verbal brain. They may not. It takes a long time to learn how to operate our amazingly complex and unrestricted quantum field generators. Parents expect to hear "mama" and "dada" within the first year after the child is born. When that doesn't happen, they begin to panic and seek professional help.

By way of explanation, consider your garden. When you buy a fruit tree at the nursery, the grower will usually tell you how long it will take for the tree to start bearing fruit. Very few trees will fruit in the first season after planting. Many trees require specific pollinators (other varieties of the same kind of tree + bees or insects) to be placed in proximity or they will never bear fruit. You accept this, put in the work, and wait patiently for years for the first signs of fruit. But no one gave you the owners' manual for your autistic child, family member, friend, colleague, or spouse. No one told you how long it would take for that amazing individual to learn how to manage language. No one told you how long it would take, if ever, for that person to vocalize coherently in your chosen language. So, you panic. In your panic, you may seek out the quickest and easiest path to what you think will be success. This path is populated by charlatans and other nefarious people who often prey upon the uninformed.

Here's how we'll fix it

In my life, my first attempts at vocal communication came in the form of echolalia. I heard, stored, and sorted words and phrases that seemed useful. These came from my primary sources of communication – the radio, TV, and my family. Most of these sources were divorced of context – I had no idea which words were appropriate to which situations. I had to learn this over time. My immediate family were well-skilled in foul-mouthed sarcasm. These were not the most appropriate sources for my echolalia. Trial and error were used to test out my new skill – resulting mostly in error.

The medical world sees echolalia as a disorder to be cured (Neely et al., 2016). Language pathologists exist to help people with problems using language. But, for neurodivergent people, echolalia is not a problem or a disorder as such. It's a way of communicating. Many autistic people do not do well with language pathologists because echolalia, for us, isn't a disorder – it's an attempt at communication. The pathologists' efforts to correct our behavior often cause more problems than they solve (Roberts, 2014). In the clinical setting, the person defining what counts as acceptable speech is all too often not the autistic person themselves. From the autistic person's standpoint, their echolalia may be perfectly well contextualized and richly significant (Seymour, 2022).

By way of continuing the example, the years between birth and puberty can be a very frustrating time for parents and autistic children. Imagine having a new roommate who doesn't speak your language and comes from a completely different culture. How do you get along? How do you set rules? How do you set anything? How do you communicate? Eventually, you each learn a bit of the other's culture and preferred mode of communication. You figure it out as you go along, together, respectfully. The same holds true when autistics (children) and non-autistics (parents) meet. For me, echolalia meant that I was pretty good at mimicry. In my multi-ethnic and multilingual melting pot of city and schools, I now had a menu of phrases in English, Spanish, German, Russian, and Armenian. I worked hard at sounding correct in each language and dialect that I repeated in response to questions and requests. Sometimes, the languages got confused in delivery, much to the endless delight of my peers.

But in my attempts to fit in socially, I found that I could use my echolalia to amuse my classmates by adding accents and flair when reading aloud in class. I could switch from my "BBC presenter voice" of my grandmother's TV programs to the "Mexican warehouseman voice" of my summer jobs with amazing agility. I had amazing oral fluency, but I had no idea what I was saying. I couldn't yet comprehend the languages I was speaking.

On the other side, when my brain is quite overwhelmed, vocal communication is impossible. Pops, clicks, and other sounds (combined with blank and panicked stares) substitute for words. This is the same today, after 50, as it was when I was young. When I was young, it just seemed weird to my peers and friends. Today, as novel vocal demand on my non-verbal system increases, I find myself sliding up the ASD severity scale as my language impairment conspires against my productivity. Indeed, studies show an inverse relationship between ASD severity scale and verbal/vocal ability (Sanz-Cervera et al., 2015).

As a result of this knowledge, I spend a great deal of time preparing for occasions that will require me to be vocally extemporaneous. In more formal settings, I often write out scripts that support my speaking and that I offer as lecture notes for the audience. In less formal settings, I may limit the amount of time that I spend engaging in the activity. I'm open and honest about what I'm doing when I'm doing it. As such, I model what the autistic experience looks like in a neurotypical environment. I also rely upon my hyper-empathy and alexithymia to "read" the room as I don't process faces in a neurotypical fashion. This keeps me from the autistic tendency to lose track of time when engaging in one's special interest (Boucher, 2001).

Such are my experiences as an autistic person. It must be noted here that on the opposite end of the verbal spectrum are the hyperlexic. Hyperlexia is a combination of advanced word-recognition skills in individuals who otherwise have cognitive, social, or linguistic disabilities, the early acquisition of reading skills without direct or explicit instruction, and a strong preference toward written material (Nation et al., 2006). Hyperlexia is strongly associated with autism, with more than 80 percent of cases co-occurring with autism (Ostrolenk et al., 2017). In school, a hyperlexic child will often score well above their grade level in oral fluency and decoding, but very low in comprehension (Cardoso-Martins and Da Silva, 2010). In other words, hyperlexic children do very well at reading individual words, but often lack the ability to comprehend the meaning of those words when collected into sentences or paragraphs. This is a significant point for educators to consider when interpreting scores on diagnostic assessments and planning interventions.

End of chapter activity

For our end of chapter activity, you will research and report on how autism is presented in academic literature. Using the suggestions from the chapter to guide your work, find and catalog between 10 and 20 articles and papers that reflect a diversity of opinion on the subject. From this information, write a short paragraph on what it means to be autistic. Here, Fromm's work on the space between having and being can inform your work. Try to incorporate aspects of place in your findings. In other words, does the presentation of autism in the research you've discovered differ in relation to the place in which it is studied?

Summary

In this chapter, we focused on what autism is, laying a foundation based both on the medical model and the social model. We saw that with most Western societies treating autism as a disorder, we must understand that framework and how autism is diagnosed and classified. Also, we began our work on the social side of autism, making our initial discoveries into the ways in which autistic people may identify. We concluded with a brief example on the differences between verbal and non-verbal, and how these concepts may be different from non-speaking.

Key vocabulary, terms, and people

- **Alexithymia.** The inability to recognize or describe one's own emotions as originating either within themselves or having been transferred to them from another source. A common, yet commonly missed, co-morbidity in autistic people.
- **Identity-first/person-first language.** Person-first language introduces a person before any description of them. Identity-first language refers to wording about a person that leads with a description of them in the context

of an identity, disability, ethnicity, gender, or other difference. Examples include terms like autistic person, trans person, or African American person.

- **Medical model of disability.** The medical model tends to emphasize biological defects and/or dysfunctions when speaking of what disability is. Within this model, the limitations disabled people experience are accounted for by reference to some biological pathology – a clinically observable impairment in bodily structure or function. The medical model does, however, recognize that functional limitations can be dependent upon a myriad of environmental factors.

- **Model of disability.** In a general sense, a model of disability aims to accomplish two goals. First, it attempts to account for what it means to be disabled. Then, it attempts to identify the causes of the disability. As such, any model should identify why it is that a person experiences the limitations associated with the disability.

- **Nosography.** In medicine, it is a description whose main purpose is enabling a diagnostic label to be put on a situation or condition.

- **Nosology.** The branch of medical science dealing with the classification of diseases.

- **Phenomenological.** Relating to the science of phenomena as distinct from that of the nature of being.

- **Social Model of Disability (SM).** The social model attempts to account for the limitations disabled people experience in terms of their social isolation, oppression, and exclusion from participation in everyday life. Within the social model, the limitations disabled people experience are caused by factors that come from outside of the person, not from their impairment or disability. In the view of those that advocate for this model, the real problems disabled people face come from the surrounding social, institutional, and physical environment with which the disabled must deal.

- **Jacques Bertillon.** French statistician and demographer. Author and creator of the Bertillon Classification of Causes of Death. The Bertillon Classification was the first classification system of diseases in which all known diseases were arranged in chapters according to their anatomical and/or pathological basis. The Bertillon Classification was the predecessor of the International Classification of Diseases (ICD).

Building background knowledge

The following titles are not required reading but will serve those who study this topic by providing valuable context and background knowledge.

Fromm, E. (1995). *The Essential Fromm: Life Between Having and Being*. Continuum.

Erich Fromm (1900–1980) was a German American psychoanalyst who highlighted the function of culture in the development of one's personality. Fromm believed that character in humans evolved as a way for people to meet their needs. Fromm's work revolved around what he believed were humanity's five essential needs: relatedness, rootedness, transcendence, sense of identity, and a frame of orientation.

This title is a posthumous collection of Fromm's unpublished lectures, interviews, and probing observations as well as key selections from his *To Have or to Be* and *The Art of Being*.

Fromm, E. (1997). *On Being Human*. Continuum.

This title is a posthumous collection of Fromm's writings and lectures on "New Humanism." Here, the odd connection between the **concepts of man** put forth by Karl Marx and the life and works of the medieval German Catholic mystic Meister Eckhart lay a foundation for the exploration of what it means to be disabled in a Western capitalist society.

Silvers, A. (2009). An essay on modeling: The social model of disability. In: D. C. Ralston and J. Ho (eds.), *Philosophical Reflections on Disability*. Springer, pp. 19–36.

This essay is a concise treatment on the war between the medical and social models of disability (Silvers, 2009).

3
When is autism?

Learning objective

With autism in mind, students will be able to reconstruct the story of humanity from the distant past until the present.

Activity

Students research and report on a time and place where relatively solitary humans seemingly saved humanity from the brink of extinction. What was it about this time and place where the traits commonly associated with autism seemed to place this group at an advantage?

Introduction

"After an exhaustive review of your case (or your child's case), we've determined that you (or they) meet the diagnostic criteria for a diagnosis of Autism Spectrum Disorder," says the doctor. These words often bring relief to autistic people or those that care for them upon receiving a formal diagnosis of ASD. They will now have greater access to supports. They will now be an official part of the autistic and disabled community.

For the self-diagnosed, the journey to self-diagnosis is quite different (Lewis, 2017). They've examined the many sources of information available on what it means to be autistic, they may have taken the many surveys that are available online, and from that information found that the traits described therein, and the scores received, describe them and their life experiences best – they're autistic (Sarrett, 2016).

Now what?

Often, they conduct internet searches to find those who might also be autistic. They look for community. They look for support. They find what the search engine algorithms return, which is not necessarily what they are looking for. Being new to the experience, they do not have a metric with which to judge the search results. Some get frustrated. Some join online communities in spaces like Facebook and Instagram. Some are welcomed in these spaces. Others, however, find that their intersectional identities clash with the dominant narratives in these spaces (Hammond, 2022). So, they keep searching.

As we saw previously, how we search the internet will impact the results we receive. As an example, type in the following query into your favorite search engine: "history of autism." You will likely find a consensus on a timeline of events (Wolff, 2004) that jumps from 1908 (autism is first described by Bleuler) to 1943 (Kanner publishes a paper) to 1944 (Asperger publishes a paper) and so on. You can go ten pages into your search (I used Bing) before concluding that the featured timeline is likely accurate. Based on your search, you may determine that Leo Kanner is the first doctor to describe what we now call autism.

Guess what? That's simply not true (Feinstein, 2011).

Let's modify our search parameters. We'll type "discovery of autism" and "Sukhareva." What did you find? Did you find Grunya Sukhareva, the actual "discoverer" of autism (Sher and Gibson, 2021)?

Grunya Efimovna Sukhareva, unfortunately, is only known in small professional circles outside of the view of Western medicine (Simmonds, 2019). For psychiatrists in Russia and the countries that formed what used to be the Soviet Union and its allies, she is the greatest authority on the topic of autism. In celebration of her pioneering work, one of the best psychiatric clinics in Russia is named after her. Indeed, the former Moscow Scientific and Practical Center for Mental Health of Children and Adolescents, which was founded in 1895, was renamed in her honor. But for most people around the world, her name is not at all familiar (Manouilenko and Bejerot, 2015).

A solid footing

The news that search results are skewed by a variety of factors is likely not new to you. Search engine results pages can be skewed by source bias, algorithmic bias, and cognitive bias (Novin and Meyers, 2017). Thus, we must be very specific when entering search terms into our favorite search tool. What we have discovered with our brief experiment is that there is a dominant narrative around discovery of autism. This narrative, if we continue along its trajectory, will necessarily bias our search for the historical roots of autism and its implications. Thus, we need to set the record straight. We need to go where the facts lead us.

This fact-based inquiry will likely trigger some uncomfortable reactions. It may outrage some. It may lead down some dark corners of our recent past. But it's necessary to cover this information. We must begin our historical inquiry on a solid footing. We must begin from the actual discovery of autism, along with the reasons why the discovery was made in the first place. From there, we will deconstruct the differences between Sukhareva's and Kanner's/Asperger's discoveries. These differences center around why the diagnosis was given and what was done with and to the autistic person after the diagnosis was delivered.

Paedology vs. scientific racism

Before listing the specific traits associated with autism as a guide to our inquiry, it is necessary to define a few terms and methods. It is also necessary to declare some limitations to our work. These limitations, as you will see, are informed by ethical scientific practice when working with human subjects in research – both the living and the deceased.

To begin, before Russia became the dominant part of the Soviet Union, Russian pedagogues, psychologists, psychiatrists, and pediatricians were hard at work studying childhood development (Minkova, 2012). The period around the beginning of the twentieth century was quite active for a study of these topics (Kirschenbaum, 2013), then called pedology or paedology (педология). Paedologists examined not only the child but the child's total context. Information from genetics certainly informed their work, but so too did the culture of the family and the local or contextual conditions. The goal wasn't necessarily to change the child, or to alter the gene pool. Quite the contrary. The goal was to create the optimal conditions whereby the child could thrive. It was hoped that schools full of thriving children would grow up to be productive members of society (Minkova, 2012).

Although the relationship between the Soviet Union and the Western powers soured quickly after the conclusion of the Second World War, thus blocking the flow of academic research and ideas between the two sides, there are legacies of the prominent paedologists to be found in Western education systems today. As an example of this, teachers are trained to use Vygotsky's Zone of Proximal Development (ZPD) in creating the perfect conditions for their students' growth (McLeod, 2012). ZPD is a perfect example of the mindset of those paedologists.

Within this context, of finding the optimal conditions within which students will thrive, Dr Sukhareva sought to understand what she called in her 1930 paper the autistic attitude. Just as modern teachers are taught to do today, she sought to get to know those in her care at a personal level. In this way, she could differentiate their experiences and achieve optimal results. They could thus learn, grow, and thrive.

Her work in the early 1920s informed the eventual publication of a list of autistic characteristics in her 1925 contribution to the book, *Questions of Pedology and Child Psychoneurology* (pp. 157–187). That contribution, titled "Schizoid psychopathy in childhood," contained the following description of the characteristics of those soon to be described as autistic children (Ssucharewa, 1926).

An autistic attitude: Tendency toward solitude and avoidance of other people from early childhood onward; avoids company with other children.

- Impulsive, odd behavior.
- Clowning, rhyming.
- Some were speaking endlessly or asking absurd questions of the people around them.
- Affective life flattened.
- Seems odd.
- A tendency toward abstraction and schematization (the introduction of concrete concepts does not improve but rather impedes thought processes).
- Lack of facial expressiveness and expressive movements.
- Mannerism; decreased postural tone; oddities and lack of modulation of speech.
- Superfluous movements and synkinesis.
- Nasal, hoarse, or high-pitched whining voice or lacking in modulation.
- Keep apart from their peers, avoid communal games and prefer fantastic stories and fairy tales.
- Find it hard to adapt to other children.
- Ridiculed by their peers and have low status.

Tendency toward automatism: Sticking to tasks which had been started and psychic inflexibility with difficulty in adaptation to novelty.

- Tic-like behaviors.
- Grimacing.
- Stereotypic neologisms.
- Repetitive questioning; talking in stereotypic ways.
- Rapid or circumscribed speech.
- A tendency for obsessive-compulsive behavior.

- Lengthy preparation and difficulty stopping.
- Pedantic, follows principles.
- Emotional outbursts.
- If interrupted becomes agitated and starts the story all over again.
- Strong interests pursued exclusively.
- Preservative interests, for example, conversation marked by repetitive obsessional themes, clings to certain themes.
- Tendency to rationalization and absurd rumination.
- Musically gifted – enhanced perception of pitch.
- Sensitivity to noise, seeks quietness.
- Sensitivity to smell.
- Onset in early childhood.
- Inability to attend normal school due to their odd behaviors.
- Intelligence normal or above normal.

Compare the above list of autistic traits to those found in the modern literature. Notice how Sukhareva's observations largely mirror DSM-V (Posar and Visconti, 2017). As we look back, how many autistic people could have been identified and helped in the West between 1925 and the early 1990s if Western doctors had access to Sukhareva's body of knowledge?

If Western doctors didn't have access to "Soviet science," from where did they get their information? That answer is simple and spans most of the search results you found earlier. Leo Kanner and Hans Asperger are seen in the West and by the search engine algorithms as the "discoverers" of autism. Most mainstream books on autism printed in the West, such as Silberman's *Neurotribes*

(2015), seem to present this view. Unfortunately, this legacy has caused untold death and suffering for autistic people.

While Sukhareva and her paedologist colleagues sought to identify autistic students to improve their outcomes, eugenicists like Asperger sought to identify them so that they could be eliminated from society and thus not corrupt the gene pool (Sheffer, 2018). Such is the nature of scientific racism (Jackson, Weidman, and Rubin, 2005). As Edith Sheffer has so accurately detailed, the autistic person was a threat to the cohesion of German society. Being solitary and independent was seen as a troublesome disability in Nazi Europe. Being autistic was not only a problem in the present tense but also represented a threat to the future of the German *volk*. The so-called racial hygiene programs (aka scientific racism) were meant to put these poor suffering autistics out of their misery. Along the way, thousands of children and adults were put to death by the state (Black, 2012).

In the Soviet context, the goals were not the elimination of the disabled but the establishment of structures and supports that were put in place to allow the person to thrive, thus assisting the collective in achieving its goals (Minkova, 2012). Within the Nazis' genocidal ideology, Asperger's work sought to ascertain if the autistic person could be cured. If the person was seen to be "high functioning," they would be institutionalized, and cures would be attempted. If the cures didn't work, the child was determined to be "low functioning." At this low end of the functioning scale, it wasn't thought that a cure was possible. The low functioning were quickly euthanized. Thus, a diagnosis in Nazi Europe could easily lead to death (Sheffer, 2018).

Lest you think that this ideology was limited to Europe, the underlying premise that informed the racial hygiene programs of the Nazis was alive and well throughout the Western world. In fact, the Nazis didn't invent racial hygiene; they imported it from the US (Black, 2012). There, it was known by another name – eugenics. California, for example, passed the Asexualization Act of 1909 (Jogoleff, 2012). Proponents of the Act believed that by sterilizing people with mental illnesses, physical disabilities, and other so-called undesirable traits, they would improve humanity (Laughlin, 1922). The low functioning in California were often confined to state-run hospitals where the sterilizations were performed. The Act and subsequent acts in support of it were finally repealed in 1979 (Whatcott, 2020). In 2021, a program to compensate survivors was created within the state's budget and administered by the California Victim Compensation Board (State of California, 2021).

Ethics and standards

With this horrific legacy in mind, we must be careful in assigning a diagnosis where none is requested. Many popular websites have written articles ascribing a diagnosis of autism or Asperger's Syndrome to various historical figures. From Thomas Jefferson, to Michelangelo, to Mozart (Applied Behavior Analysis Programs Guide, 2022), people seem eager to pick out items within the description of these famous people and note how they compare to autistic traits. Yet, as Sukhareva's work reminds us, no behavior happens in a vacuum. Place and time are highly relevant factors. Jefferson, for example, is listed as possibly being autistic because of his shyness and lack of a sociable nature. It is also noted that he disliked loud, abrupt noises. Michelangelo's obsessiveness about his work, as well as his supposed lack of friends, is how he finds himself on the list. Sir Isaac Newton's social ineptitude and fixation on solving puzzles lands him on the list.

Yet, might there be other explanations? In science, when a declaration is made, it is to the exclusion of all other explanations. To the trained eye, *Canis familiaris*, for example, is distinct from *Canis lupaster*. The common domesticated dog is indeed quite distinguishable from the African golden wolf. Michelangelo might have preferred his own company. He might have been a driven professional. These things, in and of themselves, do not amount to autism. There are no contemporary accounts provided that frame the descriptions in terms of neurotype. The descriptions are given based upon hearsay accounts, which are often highly inaccurate.

Thus, if we are to undergo a search of our genetic past to attempt to uncover the emergence of the autistic neurotype, we must frame our search objectively. In spanning millennia, we must understand the mechanics of natural selection. We must, therefore, search for autism with natural selection in mind.

Let's set up our graphic organizer

Our journey will be guided by the work of Dr Jared Reser, the originator of the Solitary Forager Hypothesis (Reser, 2011). We will also use the criteria established by Dr Grunya Sukhareva (Ssucharewa, 1926) to account for context, as well as to add precision to our descriptions.

To build our graphic organizer, we'll need four columns and eight rows. We'll title our columns in the following manner:

- trait or symptom;
- psychological consequences;
- implications for moderns; and
- implications for solitary foragers.

We'll title our rows as follows:

- high systemizing ability;
- obsessive, repetitious tendencies;
- gaze aversion and absence of shared eye contact;
- low oxytocin;
- anomalies in anterior cingulate cortex, orbitofrontal and mediofrontal cortex;
- amygdala hyperactivity; and
- hippocampal hyperactivity.

Filling in the blanks, we see from Reser's work that a high systemizing ability has the psychological consequence of the tendency to favor the exploration of non-social processes. In modern times, this may look like a person with quirky or limited subject-matter focus but having substantial knowledge and skills within that area. In ancient times, this would look like an internal drive guiding the creation or acquisition of techniques that would assist in finding food and water.

The obsessive and repetitious tendencies often seen in autistic people have as a psychological consequence a perseveration in behavior and thought (Cooper et al., 2022). This was noted by Sukhareva in her study where she noted that autistic people display preservative interests as well as conversations marked by repetitive obsessional themes. Both Reser and Sukhareva noted that modern autistic people show a need for repetitious play and sameness. This desire for order, structure, and self-regulation/self-sufficiency is how this trait might have materialized in the distant past.

A chief complaint against autistic social interactions is the lack of eye contact (Stuart et al., 2022). This gaze aversion has the psychological consequence of a reduced or non-existent attention to the faces of others. So important is this behavior to modern contexts that Sukhareva saw this as proof of a flattened affective life or a lack of emotional connectedness. This gap in connection is an unfortunate hurdle to those in modern social situations. Yet, this aversion to looking at someone directly in the eyes may be instinctual. Here, as in our past, the autistic person instinctually does not wish to challenge or provoke (Reser, 2011).

Low oxytocin levels have been linked to depression and anxiety. They have also been linked to reduced social interest, learning, and expressiveness (Dou, 2022). When Sukhareva described her autistic students as having a lack of facial expressiveness and expressive movements, of having emotional outbursts, and as being quickly agitated, she was likely observing this low hormone state. This is likely the culprit behind what Sheffer (2018) described as the Nazis' fixation on autistics lacking *Gemüt*. While there is no direct translation possible, the idea of *Gemüt* ties in with being able to connect one's spirit with the collective, or, as Reser describes, unfortunately hindered social cognition. Yet, from an evolutionary standpoint, this tendency would help in times when the environment was socially impoverished.

Modern scientists love to use their new scanning tools. Some have discovered that autistic people have a tendency toward anomalies in their anterior cingulate cortex, as well as their orbitofrontal and mediofrontal cortexes (Sha et al., 2022). The result of this can lead to a reduced desire for social learning, as well as a reduction in the need to affiliate with others. This hindered social integration that Reser (2011) noted shows up in Sukhareva's work as a tendency toward solitude as well as the avoidance of other people. This behavior was observed from early childhood onward (Ssucharewa, 1926). While modern autistic students may hate group work in school, preferring to work alone, this behavior may come from an ancient need to decrease reliance on others (Reser, 2011).

Hyperactivity within the amygdala can lead to a variety of problems. This region of the human brain manages emotional responses and states such as fear, anger, and pleasure. The psychological consequences of the potentiation of innate and conditioned fears often confound psychiatrists when their autistic patients come to them seeking relief. This can often lead to excessive anxiety and a voluntary withdrawal from social life. Night-terrors (quite common within the autistic population [Relia and Ekambaram, 2018]), or the brain's attempt to reconcile past traumas during sleep, are also linked to a hyperactive amygdala (Edwards, 2015). Yet, in the perhaps not so distant past, a hyperactive amygdala may have caused a healthy dose of caution, as well as a fear of unfamiliar people, which would have served to protect our autistic ancestors from harm (Reser, 2011). Sukhareva's note about emotional outbursts may have been an attempt at repelling the unfamiliar. Remember, our autistic ancestors would have had to survive long enough to reproduce and pass along their genes to the next generation.

When it comes to hippocampal hyperactivity, this is where the modern employment trends tend to focus. Autistics, it seems, can access contextual and episodic information at a superior level. This is evidenced in the Israel Defense Force's leveraging of autistics in their spatial intelligence efforts (Ono Academic College, 2022). Sukhareva noted this as an increased sensitivity across many perceptual domains. Indeed, my own proficiency with spatial tasks and contextual memory within the forensic analysis of images, video, and audio signals speaks anecdotally to this trait. In ancient times, the skill in tests of spatial intelligence would have enhanced one's ability to acquire and secure sources of food and water (Reser, 2011).

Now that we know what we're looking for, there are a few important issues that we will need to touch upon before starting our search.

Three important issues

1. Correlation is not causation. In causation, there is a provable relationship between variables. For causation to exist, it must exist in every case. For example, many people believe that cigarette smoking correlates to the development of cancer in humans. Cigarette smoking, in and of itself, does not cause cancer. This is because there are many cases of people living a long, smoking-filled life. To be sure, there is a strong correlation. But we can't say that smoking cigarettes causes cancer in every smoker. Again, the key phrase here is "in every situation." Correlation doesn't involve every situation,

only the data you have right now (e.g., your uncle who died of lung cancer after a lifelong smoking habit). Causation, on the other hand, involves every situation, including many situations not included in your current data. Here, we can understand that rain clouds are the direct causal link to rain… even if it hardly rains where we live.

2. Seek alternative explanations. Rather than trying to prove yourself right, try to prove yourself wrong. Consider that what you interpret as autistic behavior within a historical account of an individual or group could be a literary device utilized by the author to serve a particular end. Remember, history is written by the victors. Rarely do they speak lovingly or accurately about the vanquished or the marginalized.

3. As researchers, we are bound by ethics. Consider that researchers in most Western countries can't collect data from minors without parental or guardian consent. All participants in human subject research must give their consent to be part of a study and they must be given the relevant information necessary to give informed consent to participate. But we're not studying the living, necessarily. We're diving way back into the past. Why would the dead need to consent to be included in our research? This is where cultural sensitivities come into play. We want to respectfully investigate the past. We want to keep our own biases in check. We don't want to purposefully upset the living in our inquiries about the past.

4. Finally, it's worth noting that many areas of the world, such as sub-Saharan Africa, view autism largely as a problem of Western industrial society (Abubakar, Ssewanyana, and Newton, 2016). Thus, current research might be hard to find in these places. Plus, while an inquiry of autism in Denmark,

for example, might be looking for quirkiness, shyness, or a hyper-specialization to find potentially autistic people in their past, sub-Saharan Africa's view of autism will color your search. In the Ivory Coast, for example, the mother of an autistic child is often blamed as having done something bad that led her to be punished with a child with a "bad spirit." Seen as "evil," the autistic child is often mistreated, abused, hidden, or beaten because parents think that the autistic child deserves to be treated that way (Kobenan, 2012). Thus, a historical inquiry there would want to search not for quirky kids, but for so-called "bad spirits." Again, the inquiry begins with how autism is viewed within the context of the location being surveyed.

Here's what this might look like

My maternal grandmother's father left Scotland around the time of the Great War as part of the Crown's Red Clydeside expulsions. That side of my family had lived in Argyll since before time was time. As we now know, I'm autistic. As autism is genetic, it had to have come from somewhere. I've mentioned previously my grandmother's brother, so focusing my inquiries on her side of the family makes sense. It also helps that the Scots kept rather good genealogical records. I can dive deep into the past and read descriptions of relatives that track rather well with Sukhareva's and Reser's descriptions of the autistic experience. I can also picture ancient Argyleshire's remoteness and ruggedness as being a fit place for a solitary forager. Indeed, this might be the case, but the tribal nature of the old Scottish Clans speaks against my initial instincts. Perhaps individuals broke away from the villages. I find heads of households with a dozen children. I find siblings that died childless. I find other relatives who died during childhood.

As I gather my data, I start to see strong correlations. Certain branches of my family seem entirely more social than others. Following those who are less social backwards in time, I see fewer childbirths but longer lives. I'm not sure what to make of this odd data point yet. As we go back a millennium, I have no direct records to examine. I have histories written by victors. The modern Scottish borderlands are a mess in the period from 700 CE to 1000 CE. Danish adventurers arrived and expanded their holdings. My father's last name is a derivative of this time in history, coming originally from Kings Horik I (Hårik I) and Horik II (Hårik II) who ruled their empire in the middle part of the 800s. Were the wandering and adventuresome Danes the source of my autistic genes? Were the conquered Scots relying upon their excited autistic amygdalae to beat a path into the relative safety of the mountains?

The legends around the family structures of this time and place are quite uniform. As my grandmother shared with me, on the male side, the first-born son was to take over the leadership of the family upon the death of the father. The second-born son was to be an aide to his older brother, a vice-president of sorts. Further sons were seen as potential challengers to their older siblings and were often sent away to monasteries. Engaged in a religious vocation, it was hoped that they would not produce offspring who might challenge for leadership of the family. On the female side, daughters were often married off to form alliances. In times when no male heir was produced, the oldest daughter did assume the leadership of the family until such time as a suitable male heir was produced.

Disabled children were often left in care of the Church (Bohling, Croucher, and Buckberry, 2022). The Church might find it difficult to care for them in the big cities. They would often assign them to distant monasteries and abbeys. Monastic life would seem well suited for the autistic person: ritual, routine, quiet, and remote. Spatial intelligence would lend itself well to script copying, one of the many monastic vocations. So said my grandmother. Perhaps she was attempting to steer me to the priesthood and monastic life?

Going further back in time, author Thomas Cahill documents the time immediately after the fall of the Roman Empire when the monks of these remote abbeys helped to restart Christian civilization. He notes Saint Colmcille's work in what is now Argylleshire and the establishment of the abbey on the island of Iona. The Iona of the 500s would be considered the ends of the earth. Yet, Iona Abbey was a thriving monastic community. Its monks were credited with not only preserving important Christian texts but with single-handedly going out into the pagan world to re-establish their Church across Europe (Cahill, 1996).

Could some of these monks have been autistic? The autistic neurotype certainly lends itself to remote monastic life. What about traveling solo, far away from home, to achieve a sought-after goal? I can't help but think, what an amazing time and place to be autistic. I can't also help thinking that if it's true, that autistic people were in part responsible for saving Christianity as we know it, we should have our proper place in the Church's history – as heroes. From a Complementary Cognition standpoint (Taylor,

Fernandes, and Wraight, 2022), the Iona Abbey and the restart of Christianity helps explain how humanity evolved in diverse but complementary ways.

Let's debrief what you saw

I began my inquiry with me, an autistic person. I attempted to use family lore to trace a path backward in time to find that "first" autistic ancestor. I provided specifics as to dates and places. I offered context about how place and culture might have contributed to the success of my autistic genes being passed down to me through generations. I went back to a time and place where these traits that we now call autism seemed to help save the collective from a major calamity.

But here's where you might get tripped up. All of what was presented was anecdote. There's no mention of autism, as such, in the records of Iona Abbey. No mention of disabled abbots or monks. There's no hard science. No DNA samples to compare. And therein lies the problem. There is no genetic test currently for autism. We can't dig up old bones and check them for autistic genes. We can't even test ourselves for autism. Remember, we're still relying upon the stories and accounts of our parents and teachers to inform autism diagnoses. Nevertheless, this is all that we have currently.

So, here's how we'll fix it. We want to collect these stories. We want to fill in the blanks. We want to document our history. We want to tell our own stories. You can help us in this effort. Thus, we will collect this data. We'll look for the clues using Reser's (2011) and Sukhareva's (1926) criteria as our guide. We'll look first in our own history. Then, we'll expand further out in place and time to attempt to build a clearer picture of autism in the contexts in which we engage. If you are not autistic, you may choose to help someone close to you, a family member or student who is.

End of chapter activity

Pick a geographic location. It could be your current residence. It could be your hometown. It could be, like me, where your ancestors came from. Provide a rough outline of the history of the peoples of that place. Search, collect, and report on the time and place where relatively solitary humans inhabited or interacted with those in that space. Use your graphic organizer to help guide your inquiry and keep track of the data that you will collect.

As you build this data set, you may notice that there are times in which these solitary foragers seemingly saved their culture/country/humanity from the brink of disaster/extinction. What was it about this time and place where the traits commonly associated with autism seemed to place this group at an advantage? Why do you think that is? Given the depth of history, your response length will likely be between 1,500 and 2,000 words.

Summary

In this chapter, we focused on the when of autism. We dove further into autism's traits. We were faced with some uncomfortable truths about the diagnostic history of autism and how it has been used for evil ends. As we became familiar with the work of Dr Jared Reser, we saw how it is possible that autism has likely existed in the human genome for many tens or hundreds of thousands of years. We can imagine our autistic ancestors mixing with Neanderthal. Realizing that not enough has been written and collected about the benefits autistic people bring to our communities, we assembled a narrative of one family or group to illustrate how the autistic neurotype can be the hero in the classic hero's journey.

Key vocabulary, terms, and people

- **Complementary cognition.** The theory that combining a variety of cognitive abilities within the human collective would enable humanity to co-create superior technologies, solve problems of ever-increasing complexity, and accelerate successful and sustainable adaptation to the significant changes our species has faced over the millennia.

- **Epigenetics.** The study of changes in organisms caused by modification of gene expression rather than alteration of the genetic code itself.

- **Eugenics.** The use of procedures and policies such as selective breeding and forced sterilization to improve the genetic purity of humanity. It is also known as scientific racism.

- **Evolutionary psychiatry.** A branch of evolutionary medicine, it is an approach to psychiatry/psychopathology that attempts to use evolutionary frameworks to explain psychiatric disorders.

- **Molecular anthropology (aka genetic anthropology).** The study of how genetics has contributed to human evolution.

- **Pedology/paedology.** The study of children's development and behavior. It was largely practiced/studied in Russia/Soviet Union from approximately 1900 until 1932.

- **Johann Friedrich Karl (Hans) Asperger (1906–1980).** An Austrian physician. Best known for his 1944 paper, "Die 'Autistischen Psychopathen' im Kindesalter" [Autistic psychopaths in childhood]. His work remained largely unknown in the English-speaking world as he published in German. This changed in 1976 when Lorna Wing introduced his work and coined the term Asperger's Syndrome in her paper, "Kanner's Syndrome: A historical introduction."
- **Paul Eugen Bleuler (1857–1939).** A Swiss psychiatrist. In 1911, he introduced the concept of autistic behavior and thinking as a secondary schizophrenic symptom.
- **Leo Kanner (1894–1981).** An Austrian American psychiatrist. Best known for his 1943 paper, "Autistic disturbances of affective contact," and his 1944 paper, "Early infantile autism."
- **Karl König (1902–1966).** An Austrian pediatrician who founded the Camphill Movement in Scotland. The Camphill Movement spawned residential communities around the world that continue to provide support for people with special needs.
- **Grunya Efimovna Sukhareva (1891–1981).** A Soviet child psychiatrist. She was the first to publish a detailed description of autistic traits (symptoms) in 1925. Her paper, published first in Russian and then a year later in German, wasn't published in English until 1996. Her descriptions of autism are quite like those found in DSM-5.
- **Lev Vygotsky (1896–1934).** A Soviet psychologist/paedologist. He is known for his work on psychological development in children. His methodology around the so-called Zone of Proximal Development continues to inform educators' work to this day.

Building background knowledge

The following titles are not required reading but will serve those who study this topic by providing valuable context and background knowledge.

Black, E. (2012). *War Against the Weak: Eugenics and America's Campaign to Create a Master Race-Expanded Edition*. Dialog Press.

Chesterton, G. K. (1922). *Eugenics and Other Evils*. Cassell and Company Limited.

Sheffer, E. (2018). *Asperger's Children: The Origins of Autism in Nazi Vienna*. W. W. Norton & Company.

4
Where is autism?

Learning objective

Using one of the languages native to the many cultures across the world, students will be able to describe an authentic autistic experience in relation to that culture's place.

Activity

Students research and report on autistic people within a community somewhere in the world that is not their own. How is one recognized as autistic within that community? (e.g., how does the greater Māori community treat the Takiwatānga?) How do people behave toward them? Is the context enabling or disabling? What might you change if you could?

Introduction

Before I became aware of my system being different, my experience of what we now call autistic meltdowns and shutdowns was written off by my mental health providers as a reaction to my rather traumatic childhood. When I sought help to figure out not only why my system was behaving so erratically, and how to stop this from happening, the doctors would want to sit down for hours of talk therapy. Let's pause here for a second.

How does a non-verbal person navigate talk therapy? Pause ended. It didn't. The countless sessions didn't work. The sessions didn't work because the doctors didn't really understand me, or why I was melting down. For me, during a crisis, it was the worst possible thing. The people that were supposedly there to help had no idea how. In fairness, the doctors could only recommend therapies and strategies based upon their own education and experience. None had training on autism. Thus, none knew what to look for. They fell back upon what they knew: Western psychoanalysis.

The first of my actual shutdowns happened when I was living in Germany. My problems there, in retrospect, stemmed from my love of dancing. My alexithymic system loves dance halls, discos, raves, and other live music events. The energy is amazing. The flow states that are possible are incredible. The euphoria is endless. But my autistic sensory system also needs to rest and recharge. It needs downtime. It needs to have quiet time. If only we came with a user guide.

In the little college town of Heidelberg, in southwestern Germany, there was an amazing nightlife scene. From Wednesday night through to Sunday morning, the party seemed to go on without end. This was also the time that a now famous Austrian energy drink entered the market in Germany. I would go to work on Wednesday, then take a wee nap, have an energy drink, then off to the clubs until sunrise. A quick shower and change of clothes, plus an energy drink, and it was off to work. This would repeat each day until Sunday. Some weekends, my friends and I would jump on a train to continue the fun in a distant city. Other weekends, my girlfriend and I would take trips to historic sites.

A week in Paris. A long weekend in Budapest. Fasching in Basel. Frülingsfest. Volksfest. As we hopped on trains and buses, all of western Europe was ours to explore.

Inevitably, the cumulative effects of this non-stop lifestyle took its toll. The first shutdown I experienced terrified me. Additionally, it was the beginning of the end of my relationship with my girlfriend. To her, and to the German medical system, my symptoms and behaviors made no sense. I was clearly experiencing an alarming amount of distress, but I lacked the words to describe what was happening. At that time and place, medical science had no solutions for me. They had, however, a solution for themselves – I had to leave. There was no place in rural southern Germany for an American citizen with serious and mysterious medical issues. Their advice: go home to the US for treatment of whatever it is that was happening.

With the help of family, I was able to return to the US. Within a few weeks, I found a job as a German-language clerk for a recreational vehicle rental company close by. It was relatively low paying, but it came with a health insurance plan that covered mental health services. It was through this job that I met the friends that helped me acquire and build the Combi, mentioned previously. The Combi facilitated my wandering. It also served to take me to the dance halls at night. Having not learned the reasons why my lifestyle in Germany had caused my meltdowns and shutdowns, I repeated the same patterns of behavior that caused them to return. This time, I shut down so hard that I spent a month in hospital.

In the care of a major American health care system, I spent the better part of my twenties heavily medicated and in seemingly constant therapy. When one medication didn't work, they'd prescribe others. After a while, I had gained a significant amount of weight, a common side effect from psychiatric medications (Schwartz et al., 2004). I would still melt down, but the medications made me feel claustrophobically numb about it. The feelings gave rise to panic attacks – which, they suggested, could be treated with more medicines and therapy. As the years passed, I began to get depressed. I didn't think I would ever see a path forward into sanity and stability. I felt so broken. I felt that even the best doctors couldn't fix me, much less find out what was wrong.

I was 32 and working in the police service when things began to change. By happenstance, I was invited by a distant cousin to visit his Masonic lodge. When I entered the building, I saw amazing artwork on the walls. I was told that these were reproductions of ancient tracing boards. The guide went on to explain that in ancient times, the architects and superintendents of the work would draw their designs on such boards to better instruct an illiterate workforce. Indeed, quite often, these workers came from faraway countries to help build cathedrals and other monuments. These tracing boards were instrumental in bringing together workers from different cultures, speaking different languages, into a harmonious work force. That's how Masons saw their history (Lomas, 2011). I saw it a bit different. I saw a culture using pictograms to convey complex ideas and methods. I saw a culture that "spoke" my brain's language. I turned in my application to become a Freemason that very day.

It was there that I met a man who would set me on the correct path. He was a psychiatrist working at the county's public hospital.

As it turns out, he had a lot of experience working with autistic people. As we worked together on the tasks necessary for me to advance in Masonry, he recognized me as likely being autistic. He suggested I go to a specific office within my health plan's facilities and ask for a particular doctor that he knew well. He would call ahead and brief the doctor. All I needed do was show up. I did as I was instructed. About a month later, after that four-hour conversation mentioned previously, I had the beginnings of what is now my autism diagnosis.

All these clues adding up. All these paths converging. The answers to my auditory delay. The idea that I might be autistic. The revelation that I didn't actually need medication and could thus be released from that chemical straitjacket. Hope at last. (Author's note: there's nothing wrong with needing medicine. Yet, as my experience illustrates, there's something quite wrong with taking medication that you don't need. As always, consult your doctor and ask a ton of questions.)

I share these additional details about my life's journeys to illustrate the importance of place – the where – in one's autism journey. In Germany, I had a productive life. There, I was uniquely qualified for the roles I filled. I could work and live in both the English- and German-speaking worlds. I was huge, and could thus serve as a delivery driver and bodyguard for a female salesperson who felt in constant threat from her mostly male fitness studio customers. I didn't mind the solitude of early mornings also working as a janitor at a local pub to pay my tab. Indeed, I was productive. Yet, there was no place for me. I required too much support. The state had the option to deny me services, and it did. In America, I've had periods of time, years in fact, where I did not have a health insurance plan. Here, access to quality mental health care often comes through one's company insurance plan. Until quite recently, these were only available to the most privileged and from the most expensive insurance companies. Even with the reforms of the last ten years, access to quality mental and behavioral health services is often a luxury.

There was a time, about ten years ago or so, that I thought about leaving the US again. I considered moving to Canada, the country where my mother was born. Ordinarily, the children of Canadian migrants are offered dual citizenship and the ability to join their family back in Canada. My application was denied. With my medical history, there was a risk that I would be a burden on the national health system, and I was declared "medically inadmissible" (Wilton, Hansen, and Hall, 2017). (Note: Canada's disabled migration policies have changed since 2018.) I applied to immigrate to several countries within the British Commonwealth where I have friends and family. I thought of Norway and Denmark. No. Not a chance. All denied, and for the same reasons. This all happened before the internet and social media really took off. Anecdotal reports now inform the greater neurodivergent community that immigration officials are scanning an applicant's online presence looking for reasons to deny migration applications. Even with reforms, some places, it seems, are off-limits to the disabled.

Place and its impact

We are going to explore something quite profound in this chapter. It's something every gardener knows. Given the right conditions, plants can thrive. Given the wrong conditions, they suffer and die. Humans are no different. We require the right mix of conditions to really blossom into our true selves. Yet so many of us lack the privilege of having the right place in which to thrive.

Let's consider the example studies listed in the knowledge-building section at the end of this chapter. Within them, and those like them, researchers have found that the prevalence of autism is roughly the same throughout the world. Autism certainly isn't a "Western disorder." We've discussed the idea that what we now call autism has existed in human societies since ancient times. Thus, given natural selection and human migration, we would expect to find the autistic neurotype rather evenly disbursed around the globe. Indeed, the research shows this to be the case (Zeidan et al., 2022).

To screen for autism in toddlers, many practitioners use the Modified Checklist for Autism in Toddlers Revised (M-CHAT-R) (Pop-Jordanova and Zorcec, 2021). It's available in over 40 languages, with 16 more language versions under development. You can find it for free at mchatscreen.com. Take a moment to visit the site and view the testing instrument. Read the questions. What do you think of them? Are they relevant to you and your culture? I thought of question 13 in relation to cultures who may carry their children for most of the day. Perhaps the questions might be rephrased from "does" to "can." Nevertheless, with the availability of free screening tools, the M-CHAT-R, as well as those mentioned previously, why is it that some places are more supportive of autistics than others? What is it about a specific place that makes it easier or harder for autistic people to move beyond mere survival?

Considerations

Consider what has been shared about different cultures and spaces thus far. Cultural critiques can be triggering. When working within the space of culture, especially if the researcher is not a member of that culture, the utmost care must be taken to not tread into assumptions about how culture must be. Researchers should attempt to be as free from bias as possible, or at least aware how their own cultural assumptions could bias their inquiries.

This issue is the feature of Example study 5 (see the end of this chapter), which studied language choice in a multilingual society (Orfson-Offei, 2021). The study, with the assistance of Autism Action Ghana, found that three-quarters of the respondents (parents of autistic children) chose to use only English with their autistic children. The reasons provided varied from the advice parents received from their therapists, combined with the fact that all therapies in Ghana were available exclusively in English, plus the fear of causing further speech delay in their non-vocal children should they use more than one language in the home, as well as the belief that English will take their children further in life as compared to their own indigenous languages. Consider the implication for autistic Ghanaians. The choice to focus solely on English language instruction, made with the best intentions, may further marginalize them from their culture.

What to do about it?

The Ghanaian study raises important questions that will be the feature of the remainder of this chapter. There, parents are choosing a non-native language for their autistic children in part because of a lack of available resources in their home language. They're working with therapists who are advising them to do so. Given Lacan's theories about language's link to identity (Logan, 2022), severing the child's link to their indigenous language will have a significant impact on the development of their identity as a native Ghanaian. I see this in my own classroom where migrant students and students with migrant parents argue over a fundamental question about their own identities, for example, can one truly be Hispanic (note: their choice of identity) if one has no knowledge of Spanish (Gutierrez-Vera, 2022)?

Let's consider this information another way. In Western medicine, new doctors often recite the Hippocratic Oath when beginning their practice. They swear to uphold a list of ethical standards, the most important of which is to not harm their patients. To be sure, English is the official language of Ghana. Yet, Ghanaian therapists may be harming Indigenous cultures in suggesting that parents focus on English-only instruction. This is especially true for those whose language is currently classified as endangered (Akpanglo-Nartey and Akpanglo-Nartey, 2012).

Thus, to be a part of the solution, we will now create a matrix of support based upon our own cultural contexts. Given the diversity of scholars engaged in this work, it is hoped that this body of knowledge will eventually be used to inform the world's institutions as to what autism support and inclusion can look like in a very specific context. Here, the student can play a vital role in informing the process and helping to build a culturally appropriate body of knowledge.

Let's set up your notebook

Let's first create a general statement of what autism support looks like in our unique contexts. For me, working as a special education teacher in Los Angeles, this has two aspects. There is my work as an autistic educator and the place that I create with my students. As an autistic person outside of the classroom, there are the spaces that I inhabit – both the spaces I create for myself (e.g., my home) and those that are created by others (e.g., my work and stores).

The first aspect will feel like a mission statement. Mine looks like this:

> Dr Hoerricks (they/them) is a non-verbal autistic advocate, researcher, lecturer, best-selling author, elected official, forensic scientist, and educator. As a non-verbal autistic person who happens to be hyper-empathic and alexithymic, and who was adopted at a young age into a family with a different cultural tradition than their own, they can sympathize with a diverse range of people. That complex understanding makes its way into all the content that they create and the contexts in which they engage. Having lived and worked on three continents, engaging with people from over 40 countries, they actively work to build and sustain meaningful relationships within the communities in which they serve.

Having seen what a mission statement can look like, write yours at the top of your notes page.

The second aspect, as noted above, will likely be divided into two parts. There is the space over which you have control and the spaces over which you do not. Thus, the first part can feature a list of supports that you need and have been able to provide for yourself. Remember, everyone needs supports and structure. What does yours look like? Now move to the spaces in which you inhabit – work, school, shopping, and so on. What's there that you rely upon to function? What could be added, subtracted, or modified to help you thrive?

Now that we've grounded ourselves, let's create a graphic organizer to help us collect and organize the information we will gather. To do this, we'll borrow from instructional differentiation methodology. The essence of the instructional practice of differentiation is the individualized adjustment of four curriculum-related components – **content** (what people learn), **process** (how people make sense of the content), **product** (how they demonstrate their learning gains), and **affect** (the climate of the learning environment). These are based upon three categories of needs: **readiness**, **interest**, and **learning profile** (Gross, 1980).

Thus, our columns can be created from the four curriculum-related components as well as the three categories of needs. Our rows will be created from the contexts in which we engage. From there, we can survey our environment and fill in the cells with what we discover.

Some things to watch for

This first exercise, collecting information from the world around you, will serve as practice for the chapter's activity. As you begin to examine your own context, pay close attention to the perceptions, feelings, and attitudes of those involved in creating the spaces, delivering services, and supporting people. Here's an example of how this might look.

1. In my workplace, I am not responsible for creating the spaces in which I primarily engage. The school district sets policies that are reflective of federal, state, and local laws. The administration provides oversight to ensure that these policies are enacted. As an Inclusion Specialist, I work in classrooms in which I am not the primary teacher. Within that space, I am an advocate and supporter of not only the students on my caseload, but all students in the class. Occasionally, I will disagree with a direction or method employed by the general education teacher. How I handle that disagreement can affect the climate of the classroom. I must carefully manage perceptions and feelings, all the while ensuring the best possible result for students. Thus, in relation to this aspect, what are the things that are working and what could be improved? Again, here I'm not focused on myself as an autistic person but as one who is supporting students with a diverse range of needs.

    As an Inclusion Specialist, I must absorb the curricular content and reframe it for each student in the class. To do this, I must know how each student will process this content and where they might get tripped up. I must devise an appropriate way for the student to deliver the product, to demonstrate their mastery of the subject matter. I must also ever be mindful of the climate of the classroom. This is where the Zone of Proximal Development (ZPD) is quite helpful. If I apply too little rigor, students will get bored. Behaviors will be affected. On the other side of the ZPD, too much rigor can trigger those with or at risk for emotional and behavioral disorders. Again, behaviors will be affected. It's a delicate balance to keep all this working across a classroom population of 20–30 students.

2. I am aware that the culture of American education is founded in market capitalism. The foundations of the free public school were firmly rooted in the business problem of the mass production of workers (Cohen, 1976). Here, the Protestant work ethic (Ramírez et al., 2010) was combined with management consulting and behaviorism to produce instructional designs that favor the emic over the etic. In other words, good students are productive students. Good students are those that produce the desirable grades and scores.

Here, the autistic student may only want to read about and study the AC Shelby Cobra 427 race car. Their teacher, on the other hand, may be required to have them focus on Romeo & Juliet or A Raisin in the Sun. In many modern American classrooms, where Taylorism is often mixed with Pavlovian behaviorism to produce standardized graduates, autistic students do not generally thrive. Their solitary forager instincts often drive them toward their own unique interests. Here, in this context, I have an uncomfortable choice. Am I an agent of the system? Do I go along with the flow and ensure that students produce according to the state's aims? Am I an advocate for systems change? Do I do what is in the best interest of the student and their family even if it undermines the system or my employer's goals? Such is the dilemma of the modern special education teacher.

3. The other aspect of my workplace involves me as a non-verbal autistic employee. Again, I'm not responsible for

creating the environments in which I work. I'm not shy about letting people know that I am autistic. I think most of my colleagues know by now. All my students do. Yet, much of the programming that goes on fails the "windows and mirrors" test. In other words, most of the time I must engage within a place that was not organized with someone like me in mind. I don't see myself and my needs reflected in the standard professional development offerings. Additionally, at my level, I lack the power or privilege to affect significant change. Thus, the context is rather disabling. I come home each day positively drained, completely out of spoons. This affects my decision making when asked to volunteer for afterschool projects and programs. My lack of participation in extracurricular activities may be perceived by others negatively, which can impact my career trajectory. Thus, I must be extremely careful how I manage my response to each request.

4.   Given the amount of energy that it takes to get through my day in a place and within a system that was not designed with me in mind, I need a significant amount of time to recharge each evening so that I have the energy to do it all again the next day. I think about this in relation to conversations with parents of autistic students. They often relate how their child is reported to be just fine at school but will melt down upon coming home. I relate my own story, the need to recharge, and the fact that their child probably doesn't feel safe enough at school to display that level of emotional intimacy. So, they struggle through the day and let it all go at night. It's not healthy.

Once we've created the matrix and framing, we can begin to think about these issues in other contexts.

Let's debrief what you saw

I related my own contextual information as well as how my actions might be perceived by those without an awareness of what it means to be neurodivergent in a neurotypical world. I didn't separate myself from the environment but featured my own unique needs as a part of the whole. I briefly explained what I needed to do right for those in my care, as well as what I needed to do to care for myself. I also presented some of the questions I face each day as I balance identity and activism. In this way, you get a unique view of what my context looks like.

End of chapter activity

Now, we will do this exercise again. This time, we'll use what we learned to study a population that is not our own. If you are unsure where to start, there are several example studies for you on pages 110–111. This population may share our language, or it may not. We will want to know how is one recognized as autistic within that community? How are autistic people of all ages treated there? Is the context enabling or disabling? And finally, what might we change, if we could?

Here's where we might get tripped up

You may choose to study the autistic population of a country that does little to nothing for its autistic people. Thus, there may be no studies or anecdotes from which to draw. You may not immediately know how many autistic people there will be in such countries. There may even be a language barrier. Not to worry, there are ways around these issues. Plus, gathering information about such contexts will be of great value in the overall conversation about how best to support autistic people. You may even choose to advocate for the needs of the people you discover along the way.

Some helpful fixes

If you are studying a country that does not have figures on its autistic population, we can make a few assumptions. If we take the prevalence rate for autism in general as 1:54, then we can produce a percentage of 1.85 percent of a given population. We can multiply that number by the total population to get the approximate size of the country's autistic population. For example, Myanmar does not have a comprehensive count of its autistic residents. Thus, with a population of 54.05 million people, we would expect that there will be close to a million autistic people there. 54.05m × 0.0185 = 999,925. Knowing nothing about their dispersal among the country, we might choose to drill down to a few big cities to approximate the density there. Or you can choose the largest city. In this case it's Yangon (Rangoon). Yangon's 7 million population should feature about 130,000 autistic people. 7m × 0.0185 = 129,500.

Continuing with our example of autism in Myanmar, we will encounter a problem of language. Here, Google Translate can help. If we encounter research written in Burmese, we can copy entire paragraphs and paste them into Google Translate's search fields. Here's where we might encounter problems as the perception of autism in Myanmar may be significantly different than our own. Here's an example of a paragraph lifted from a news article on autism from a local news site (Htoo, 2019):

အော်တစ်ဇင် ဆိုတာ ဉာဏ်ရည်မဖွံ့ ဖြိုးမှုဇာဂါ တစ်နည်းအားဖြင့် တဈ မသန်မစွမ်းဖြစ်ခြင်းတစ်မျိုးပါပဲ။ ဒီလို ဖြစ်သူတွရဲ့ ဇာဂါ လက္ခဏာဟာ အလွန်ပဲ ကျယ်ပန့်ပြီးကွဲပြားမှုရှိပါတယ်။ သူတို့ လဧ တွကေို သာမန် ပုံပန်းသဏ္ဍာန်နဲ့ ကြည့်ပြီးသတ်မှတ် လို့ မရပမေယ့ သူတို့ တွဟာ မွေးလာကတည်းက ဉာဏ်ရည်မဖွံ့ ဖြိုးဘဲ စကားပြာ ဆိုမှု အခက်အခဲတွ ခြင်း၊ ပေါင်းသင်းဆက်ဆံမှု မပျိုင်ခြင်း၊ လူတွ နဲ့ မိတ်သဟာဖွဲ့ မှ မလုပ်တတ်ခြင်း၊ အာရုံကြာ ချုပ်ယွင်းမှုကြောင့ ခန္ဓာကိုယ် လုပ်လုပ်ရှား ရှားမဖြစ်ခြင်း၊ သာမန်လူလို ပုံမှ ပြောဆိုမှုမ ရှိပဲ ပုံမှန်အားဖြင့် တိတ်ဆိတ်နတေတ်ကပြါတယ်။.

Google translates that paragraph as:

Autism is a type of intellectual disability. The symptoms of these people are very wide and varied. They can't be identified by looking at their normal appearance, but since they were born, they have not developed intelligence and have difficulty speaking. Inability to socialize; Not making friends with people, Immobility of the body due to nerve damage; They are usually silent without acting like normal people.

We don't have to agree with this definition to do our analysis. We can pick through the available information to find our data points. We can find what people learn and know about autism in Myanmar (**content**), how people make sense of the content (**process**), how this **content** and **process** is operationalized within Burmese culture (**product**), as well as the climate of Burmese culture for autistic people (**affect**). Through it all, we can discover if Burmese culture is **ready** and **interested** in **learning** about its autistic population and the many ways in which it can be assisted. Tragically, if we dive deeper into the example, we find that the new government in Myanmar is actively persecuting the disability activist community (Yeung, 2021). Thus, while groups like Save the Children risk their lives to help in such a hostile place, one is left to wonder how the average autistic person and their family can possibly lead anything close to a normal life in the face of such hostility.

Given the sometimes-horrific nature of what we may find, including our own reactions may help to clarify the narrative we'll create. If, for example, autism is still seen as an intellectual disability, then there may be a tremendous stigma to being autistic in Myanmar. Adults may find it even harder to find their place in Burmese society given the current volatile nature there. The absolutes given in the definition may serve to pre-bias relationships and job opportunities. After all, would you want to employ someone who is unable to socialize? Further still, given the government's position as regards activism of any kind, would you want to employ someone who may be tied to a group that is actively opposed to the current regime?

Thinking back again to Lacan and the search results from Myanmar, the declarative statements about something so fundamental to identity as autism are shocking to me. I so vehemently disagree with their assertions. Yet, this news story was among the top ten search results I found when looking for information on autism in Myanmar. Given the published information about how a Google search works (Alphabet, 2022), Google's algorithms believed that the article was within the ten most relevant stories related to autism in Myanmar. Again, when doing this kind of work, one must be prepared to be shocked with what one finds.

Now it's your turn

Considering what we've just covered, construct a graphic organizer, research an autistic population somewhere in the world, and create a brief narrative about your findings and recommendations (1,500–2,000 words). Try to include how you feel about what you've discovered as a part of your narrative.

Summary

In this chapter, we focused on the "where" of autism. We dove further into the autistic experience. We were faced with some uncomfortable truths about how autism is viewed around the world. We became familiar with some tools to help us in our inquiries. Continuing in the realization that not enough has been written and collected about the benefits autistic people bring to our communities, we assembled data and a narrative of one culture's view of autism. We can offer our new information and insights to inform the larger conversation about how place, and one's relationship to place, can impact our experience of autism and autistic identity.

Key vocabulary, terms, and people

- **Emic and Etic.** Emic is a term from cultural anthropology that has come to stand for the ambition to establish an objective and scientific approach to the study of culture. Etic, on the other hand, has come to stand for the goal of understanding the world or a culture according to the points of view of a studied population. The comprehension of these terms and the discourses that flow from them help students to grasp the struggle between the two sides in defining autism and the appropriate paths for including autistic people within a particular culture.

- **2 Thessalonians 3:10 (KJV).** "For even when we were with you, this we commanded you, that if any would not work, neither should he eat." A version of this sentence appears in Vladimir Lenin's 1917 work, *The State and Revolution*. Lenin explains there that in socialist states, only **productive individuals** should be allowed to access **the articles of consumption**. This verse forms the foundation of the so-called Protestant work ethic.

- **Vladimir L. Durov (Владимир Леонидевич Дуров) (1863–1934).** A Russian circus performer and animal trainer turned behavioral scientist. His work on behavioral training was first featured at a 1919 conference titled, "The mental influence on the behaviour of animals." Unlike Pavlov, whose work focused on conditioning a response in animals, Durov believed that his mental energy could be leveraged to command animals to his will. This mind-control/telepathy work and research would be a feature of the Soviet and American intelligence services for decades. The American side of this type of research was the feature of the 2004 book and 2009 movie, *The Men Who Stare at Goats*.

- **Aleksei Kapitonovich Gastev (Алексей Капитонович Гастев) (1882–1939).** A Russian revolutionary, labor theorist, activist, writer, and poet. He brought the concepts of Taylorism to the Soviet Union. He incorporated the concept of **setting** (установка) to scientific management to perfect the environment where labor is performed. This **setting**, this **place**, is inclusive of the interchangeable worker. In the **setting**, the worker is conditioned to optimal performance.

- **Jacques Marie Émile Lacan (1901–1981).** A French psychoanalyst. He is often referred to as "the French Freud." He and his work are quite significant within the history of psychoanalysis. His teachings and writings have influenced how national health services, as well as individual practitioners, frame and care for autistic people in clinical settings around the world. His work, like that of Erick Fromm, has much to say about the concept of autistic identity (what it means **to be** autistic). His thoughts on language's tie to identity can inform the discussion of the experience of non-verbal populations.

- **Ivan Petrovich Pavlov (Ива́н Петро́вич Па́влов) (1849– 1936).** A Russian physiologist known for his work in classical behavioral conditioning. He won Russia's first Nobel Prize for his work on the conditioning of the gastric functions of dogs. His work on conditioning continues to inform education policies and practices around the world.

- **Frederick Winslow Taylor (1856–1915).** An American mechanical engineer. As one of the first generation of management consultants, he is widely known for his methods to improve industrial efficiency and standardize performance in the workplace. In 1911, he published his techniques in *The Principles of Scientific Management*. Today, scientific management is sometimes referred to as Taylorism.

Building background knowledge

The following titles are not required reading but will serve those who study this topic by providing valuable context and background knowledge. The sample studies are provided to inform the discussion in this chapter.

Arendt, H. (1958). *The Origins of Totalitarianism*. 2nd ed. Schocken Books.

Arendt's expanded revision to her first book frames the study of mass movements and dominant ideologies in the context of the study of the two major totalitarian political movements of the recent past. The book clarifies why marginalized and minority populations are often targeted for maltreatment by government policies.

Arendt, H. (1970). *On Violence*. Harcourt Brace Javanovich.

Arendt's classic work frames power, strength, force, authority, and violence in a way that helps the reader understand how governments and other centers of power influence a person's experience of place and culture.

Hardwick, L. (2021). *Disability and the Church: A Vision for Diversity and Inclusion*. InterVarsity Press.

This book from "the autism pastor" clarifies the ideologies that are often used to exclude or further marginalize the disabled within religious communities. His work offers a vision for unity and inclusion within a Church body that does not require uniformity.

Example study 1: Arora, N. K., Nair, M. K. C., Gulati, S., Deshmukh, V., Mohapatra, A., Mishra, D., Patel, V., Pandey, R. M., Das, B. C., Divan, G., and Murthy, G. V. S. (2018). Neurodevelopmental disorders in children aged 2–9 years: Population-based burden estimates across five regions in India. *PLoS Medicine*, 15(7), e1002615.

Example study 2: Juneja, M., Mishra, D., Russell, P. S., Gulati, S., Deshmukh, V., Tudu, P., Sagar, R., Silberberg, D., Bhutani, V. K., Pinto, J. M., and Durkin, M. (2014). INCLEN diagnostic tool for autism spectrum disorder (INDT-ASD): Development and validation. *Indian Pediatrics*, 51(5), pp. 359–365.

Example study 3: Sun, X., Allison, C., Wei, L., Matthews, F. E., Auyeung, B., Wu, Y. Y., Griffiths, S., Zhang, J., Baron-Cohen, S., and Brayne, C. (2019). Autism prevalence in China is comparable to Western prevalence. *Molecular Autism*, 10(1), pp. 1–19.

Example study 4: Tuman, J., Roth-Johnson, D., Baker, D. L., and Vecchio, J. (2008). Autism and special education policy in Mexico. *Global Health Governance*, 2(1). Available at: ghgj.org/Tuman_Autism.pdf (accessed 13 August 2022).

Example study 5: Orfson-Offei, E. (2021). Autism spectrum disorder and language choice in Ghana. *Pragmatics and Society*, 12(2), pp. 288–308.

5
Who is autistic?

Learning objective

Given the DSM's dominance in the Western world, students will be able to evaluate how place influences who is considered to be autistic.

Activity

Students research and report on the path to the autistic identity in their community and contrast those findings with the path in another place in the world.

Introduction

Growing up in the eastern part of Los Angeles County, I had to take people's word that the stars came out at night. The geology of the area meant that the daily marine layer would combine with the thick blanket of smog to conspire against any real view of the sky. Day or night. We were told by our teachers that the area has always suffered from such air quality issues (Masters, 2013). In school, we would hear about the stars and planets. We would learn their names. I was happy to study these topics because for some reason, still unknown to me, I was fascinated with astronomy in general, and the planet Mars in particular. You might call it one of my special interests. It still is.

With the help of teachers, family, and friends, I learned that the planet that we now call Mars was first thought to be the Sumerian god of wars and plagues, Nergal (De Blasio, 2018). Later, when the early Greek civilization began to examine the night sky, they believed the planet to be Pyroeis ("fiery one") (Jones, 2006) – the god of the wandering star (Atsma, 2017). They later changed the name to Ares, their god of war (Graf, 2015). Ancient Chinese astronomers saw the planet and named it Fire Star (火星) (Dubs, 1958). When the Romans came along, they seemingly built on the theme of naming the planet after war gods and named the planet after their war god, Mars (Evans, 1998).

As I got older, I learned that Mars (aka the Red Planet) got its association with war due to the composition of its soil. When the sunlight reflects off its iron oxide dirt, the planet appears red to observers. Red, we were told, is the color of anger and war in many cultures. As a kid, I just accepted what I was told as fact. Mars was Mars, the Red Planet, and that was that. I never thought to question it at all.

You can make the reasonable assumption that my interest in Mars might coincide nicely with my interest in science fiction. *Star Wars* came out when I was six years old. The 1970s and 1980s were full of interesting sci-fi movies. *Star Trek* re-runs were a hit in my house as well. Additionally, my local library had a wonderous variety of science fiction comics and magazines from the 1950s to 1970s to fuel my interest. Their artwork was amazing. The few words I knew helped me to comprehend the content that the pictures were sharing. When the words were beyond me, my imagination created its own story around the characters, actions, and locations. I could look at the same comic day after day and create new stories around the same pictures to keep me entertained. There's an amazing theater in my brain.

Fast forward a few decades to my emergence as a reader. I happened to be browsing through a used book store when I saw a tattered old paperback. I don't know why it caught my eye, but it did. Perhaps, its cover, reminiscent of those old comics of my youth, was what drew my attention. Nevertheless, I paid 50 cents for Edgar Rice Burroughs' *A Princess of Mars*. As I began to read the book, a concept presented itself that shook the foundations of what I thought I knew about the Red Planet. You see, although Rice's work is fiction, he presented his readers with a profound lesson on identity. The people who inhabited Mars weren't Martians, as I had learned from the Looney Toons' Marvin the Martian. No, they were Barsoomian (Roy, 1976). Their name for their planet was Barsoom. Later, reading another book in the Barsoom series, I learned that Barsoom is a word made from the word *bar*, meaning planet, and *soom*, their word for eight. This reflected the Barsoomian view of Barsoom as the eighth astronomical body within the inner solar system, kind of like our view of Earth as the third rock from the sun. It blew my mind to consider that from their culture's founding until we encounter their story, the Barsoomians have had no contact with Rome or its gods. Thus, why would they choose a deity from another planet to identify their planet and people? It sounds silly now, but it was a profound moment for me.

I began to question all that I knew about names and places. I became fascinated with etymology. It became another of my academic special interests. I learned that the Scotland of my ancestors was not Scotland at all, but quite the mash-up of tribes whose associations shifted quite frequently. Scotland was the anglicized version of Scoti, the name given to the people who lived there by the Romans. The Roman Empire being quite dominant, it stuck (Kelti, 1881). It seems the Romans just went about naming things, places, and objects that didn't belong to them.

Where else, I wondered, might this phenomenon occur? What other names did I have all wrong? I knew from my German friends that their homeland was called Deutschland. As with Scotland, the Romans had assigned a name to an area and a people. This time, Germania was the name given to the tribes east of the Rhine river. The Deutsche, the people that live in Deutschland, have been calling themselves by that name from at least the eighth century. Deutsche, I learned, means ethnic, native, or the people. It's a way of saying, "us folk," that's more inclusive of the entirety of the population than using the Roman name for a portion of the overall population (Fulbrook, 2019). The French and Spanish names for Deutschland, *Allemagne* and *Alemania*, respectively, again reference a small confederation of tribes located near France and Switzerland. Those names are not at all inclusive of the entirety of the population.

Thus began my early work on identity. It was quite a profound revelation to find that the names I had spent so much time learning were largely imposed upon peoples and areas by conquering empires. Those original Roman names were further changed when the British Empire began to dominate the world. Growing up in an English-speaking country, these names were anglicized, or made English. My name, James, we are told, comes to English from Hebrew. There, it's *Ya'aqov* (Jacob). As I started to get annoyed at the fact that the Romans and the English seemingly changed the names of everything to suit themselves, I was told that most cultures do the same thing to make words more understandable in their own language. Jacob in Danish works fine, as there are common pronunciation rules. But it doesn't work well in Cymru (Wales), where it is *Iago* (yá-go). Wait… if *Cymru* is the Cymric word for Wales, why don't we all just call the country Cymru out of respect for the Cymry?

Taking us back to the study of autism, it's important to remember that the term autism ("selfism") was given to us by the original doctors who were studying our forebears. They were examining this group of exceptional people, attempting to classify what was atypical about them to correct what these doctors viewed as disordered or in need of support (Ssucharewa, 1926). There was no spectrum. There was no diversity. There was only the binary, ordered or disordered, normal or abnormal. They had to give this selfism a name, and then classify its traits/symptoms to assist them in restoring these people to what they believed to be a proper order based within their culture's language, norms, and needs.

Metaphysics

The further I dove into this study, the more I wondered about the type of education these doctors and scientists received. I wondered at these classifications and the big Latin words and foreign-sounding phrases that I found when I read their works. I researched the types of classes and schools available at the time. I found the so-called Classical Curriculum and the Seven Liberal Arts and Sciences. I saw a heavy reliance on the classics, the type of thought that is now collected in the 54 volumes of the *Great Books of the Western World*. As it relates here, I found Aristotle and his *Metaphysics*. Working forward from that point, I found scholars like Emerson White (White, 2013). These scholars created and administered the first colleges in the West. These administrators and pedagogues profoundly influenced how the generation of scholars that first categorized autism viewed the world. Like a method actor researching a character ahead of performing, I wanted to know the motivation as well as the knowledge base possessed by the founders of this classification system we now have.

In his 1886 work, *Elements of Pedagogy*, White noted that the authors of the classics of the West had observed that the human intellect seemed to quickly pass from personal judgment to universal facts. In a very detailed way, White attempted to decode Aristotle's *Metaphysics* for the modern student (modern in 1886). Conception, he said, takes the individual metaphysical concepts of sense and experience and forms general concepts, under which all objects are then classified. Collective judgment first distinguishes, then confirms, the common characteristics of objects and the similarity or difference of these concepts. Reason, he noted, then decodes these facts of judgment, and by induction reaches universal facts that understand and explain them. When such a universal fact is reached, and the included facts are arranged under it, the result is science (i.e., knowledge reduced to system). It was his opinion that there may be as many sciences as there are universal facts under which the related knowledge may be classified and arranged.

White (2013) was commenting on how scientists could use this common system to work both collaboratively and across disciplines. In *Metaphysics*, Aristotle wrote that in our common observations, our minds perceive only the more obvious qualities and relations of objects, and the resulting concepts are the basis of the facts of common knowledge. In its scientific phase, observation discriminates more acutely and perceives the less obvious, but often the more important attributes of objects and the resulting sharply defined concepts are the basis of scientific facts.

Facts, I learned, are different than truths. According to *Metaphysics*, facts are measurable, observable, reliable, and falsifiable. Truth, on the other hand, comes from a feeling or a belief. For example, I can stand outside in Los Angeles on a given day in August. I can measure the temperature. It might be 105 degrees Fahrenheit. If you are there with me, with similar instruments, you can repeat my experiment and achieve the same or similar results. Conversely, I may be wrong in my measurements. You may find that the temperature is only 95 degrees, thus falsifying my measurements. I check my equipment and determine it to be faulty and reconduct my measurement. This is how science works. Through it all, however, the truth of the matter is… it's hot outside. Hot is not quantifiable in and of itself. As an autistic person with sensory issues, and having erythromelalgia co-morbid, anything over 65 degrees is hot to me.

Thinking back to my former career, the basic inductions of forensic science differ from the inductions of common sense in the degree of acuteness and energy of the reasoning power required. Thus, scientific thought is, as White (2013) noted, characterized by closer observation, wider comparison, sharper analysis in conception, more accurate judgment, and more careful induction than commonly thought. In the analysis of modern autism research, at best the researchers engaged in inductive reasoning – evaluating observances in relation to claims. Mostly, however, they're engaged in abductive reasoning – taking their best shot as they work with small and convenient sample sizes. When this abductive reasoning leaps from biased theoretical constructs, problems can and do occur.

It should, however, be observed that these two phases of thought involve the same processes and the activity of the same mental powers. This fact is made evident if we compare the mental processes involved in the concepts, facts, inductions, and classifications that make up our common knowledge of plants, with those involved in the scientific concepts, facts, inductions, and classifications included in the science of botany. Our common knowledge sees a house plant, notices its color and the shape of its leaves and understands it to be English ivy. The science of botany, on the other hand, knows it as *Hedera helix*. Botany classifies *H. helix* thus (Metcalfe, 2005):

- Kingdom: Plantae;
- Clade: Tracheophytes;
- Clade: Angiosperms;
- Clade: Eudicots;
- Clade: Asterids;
- Order: Apiales;
- Family: Araliaceae;

- Genus: Hedera; and
- Species: *H. helix.*

Thinking in this way, in my former career as a forensic multimedia analyst, I regularly engaged in vehicle make/model determinations. Investigators often needed to know just what kind of vehicle was depicted within a piece of surveillance video. There, within my inquiry, I would classify the objects of my observation in a more detailed fashion, moving from "object is likely vehicle" to a very specific make/model/year/trim based on class characteristics:

- Object: vehicle;
- Make: Honda;
- Model: Fit;
- Year: 2016;
- Trim: EX; and
- Color: for example, Crystal Black Pearl or Smart Black.

I would then move to attempting to identify individualizing characteristics to link a specific vehicle to a specific person, location, and/or event.

But, as White (2013) noted, the elementary facts of science do not constitute science itself. What is further needed is that deeper insight of reason which can discern those universal facts and principles that comprehend and explain all related knowledge, thus determining and making possible its orderly classification and systematic arrangement.

But doctors and researchers should not stop with the general facts that make science possible; rather they should seek to go back to those causative energies and controlling laws that produce and explain all events and phenomena. In my previous employment, the investigators did not want to guess at the amount of damage caused by a vehicle collision (abduction) but wanted it calculated and quantified by physics and calculus (deduction). Investigators within the justice system should want to get the facts of their inquiries correct. After all, a person's life and liberty are at stake. Thinking along these lines, shouldn't those who study and work with autistic populations operate under the same premise?

Autism research generally starts out in the right direction. This pursuit of causative energies and controlling laws so often turns to drive the study of autism in the direction of cures and therapies (Rutter, 1996), a direction that most autistics do not support (Pellicano, Dinsmore, and Charman, 2014). With all this effort, there is still disagreement over who exactly is autistic. Remember, first I was just shy and a bit weird. Then, I had an identifiable problem, Sensory Processing Disorder. I also had Asperger's Syndrome/Disorder. Still me. Same person. The doctors simply found a way to classify me according to newly acquired information. The system then changed how it wanted to classify me. It made the decision to ditch the individual diagnoses and classify me as a person with Autism Spectrum Disorder. I went to bed one day having Asperger's and sensory issues. I woke up the next day autistic. After the switch in the DSM, there was no more mention of my sensory issues in my medical file. Now, with the newest changes to the DSM, DSM-5-TR, will the system revoke my classification? The jury's still out on that.

Who are autistics?

With my own journey through the diagnostic slalom course in mind, just who is autistic? How are we to know an autistic person when we encounter them? Here, we go into contentious territory. When the APA transitioned from DSM-IV to DSM-5, they created a new category from what used to be Autism, Autistic Disorder, and Asperger's Disorder. They also included some of Pervasive Development Disorder-Not Otherwise Specified (PDD-NOS) and some of the sensory processing disorders. With DSM-5, they decided to consider the entire group a "spectrum" of conditions. Thus, with DSM-5, it became Autism Spectrum Disorder (Mintz, 2017). I can recall the conversations with my care providers around this time. There was nothing for either my doctors or me to do. It was just a switch of the codes back then.

The new diagnosis came with three levels of severity. As Autism Spectrum Disorder was defined, there were "clusters of symptoms." There were issues with social interaction, social engagement, awkward social reading, social cues, preoccupation with unusual interests, and/or repeating words. The APA believed that there were two separate dimensions of the autism spectrum, so the criteria set was reformulated with these dimensions in mind. With this reformulation, they came up with a new assessment algorithm (McPartland, Reichow, and Volkmar, 2012).

The challenge then became the huge amount of interest in autism that was generated due to what appeared to be an explosion in cases of Autism Spectrum Disorder (Isaksen et al., 2013). There was the issue of lumping previous cases into the new diagnosis, and the fact that clinicians were recognizing or diagnosing it more. Additionally, there was a belief at the APA that autism was being over-recognized due to clinicians not strictly following the guidance (Elemy, 2022). Several studies examined the inter-rater reliability of the diagnostic criteria (Rice et al., 2022).

In the interim, the APA has been examining the diagnostic criteria sets, noting that the prevalence often depends upon how the clinician constructs the criteria set. For example, if you have a set of criteria that requires a positive result on five out of ten criteria, and you were to reduce the requirement to only three out of ten, the prevalence will go up a lot. If you were to require eight out of ten, you would shrink the prevalence. When the APA reformulated the autism criteria set for DSM-5-TR, it appears that they wanted to make sure that the new criteria set was conservative and that the explanations for the set were crystal clear. In doing so, less is left open to interpretation or manipulation in the new diagnostic criteria and guidance.

Again, the prevalence of diagnoses is often determined by the diagnostic structure, and with DSM-5 the APA believed that the criteria allowed too much interpretation by clinicians. The DSM-5-TR now includes the words "all of the following" before the criteria to ensure that all are being met (APA, 2022). Consequently, this may result in fewer diagnoses. Does the APA think fewer diagnoses are a good thing? Will the diagnosis rate drop? Will prevalence decline? Time will tell.

Do the APA's diagnostic criteria define who may be autistic?

Remember, to meet diagnostic criteria for ASD according to DSM-5-TR, a person must have persistent deficits in each of three areas of the listed social communication and interaction (group A) and **all four** types of restricted and/or repetitive behaviors (APA, 2022). That's a tough ask.

Bear in mind, the system will only consider a person autistic if they demonstrate to the satisfaction of the evaluators:

- persistent deficits in social communication and social interaction across multiple contexts (group A);
- restricted, repetitive patterns of behavior, interests, or activities, as manifested by all the following:

  o stereotyped or repetitive motor movements, use of objects, or speech;
  o insistence on sameness, inflexible adherence to routines, or ritualized patterns of verbal or non-verbal behavior;
  o highly restricted, fixated interests that are abnormal in intensity or focus; and
  o hyper- or hypo-reactivity to sensory input or unusual interest in sensory aspects of the environment.

When it comes to severity or so-called functioning levels, evaluators often rely upon the Childhood Autism Rating Scale (CARS) when assessing children (Flores-Rodríguez, Ceballos, and Albores-Gallo, 2022). For adults, a more subjective set of surveys are given to attempt to ascertain how much the deficits and behaviors impact the person's life.

- Level 1: Requires Support.

- Level 2: Requires Substantial Support.

- Level 3: Requires Very Substantial Support.

Again, the DSM offers evaluators no advice in assessing or suggesting the types of support that autistic individuals may need. Neither does it speak to the places in which support might help. For example, I often need support with school situations. Yet, I do just fine at home. For others, their experiences might be the opposite. Some may do well with their academic subjects but struggle with social situations. Remember, if you've met one autistic person, you've met one autistic person… once.

Additionally, the support or functioning level that a person is assigned when they're first assessed can change as they age. Access to supports that help them develop and refine their skills can change their need for those supports over time. Anxiety, depression, or other emotional issues common among autistic people can also change, increasing or decreasing in severity.

Yet, assigning people to one of the three levels of autism is part of the process. For educators and other support staff, they are useful for recommending the services and supports that would serve them best in a particular context (Lodi-Smith et al., 2019). As generic as the level descriptions are, they can't account for an autistic person's unique personality and behaviors. Thus, it's incumbent upon service providers (e.g., doctors and special education teachers) to tailor the support and services they receive to their specific situation, and then revise the recommendations at least annually.

For those areas served by the ICD, the change to ICD-11 was made to move it closer to the DSM. For autism within the ICD, there's autism, autism with or without intellectual disability, and autism with or without problems of language/communication. This breaks down to the six categories we saw previously.

From the standpoint of the current science, as defined by the ICD or the DSM, one is autistic if one is found to meet the ever-shifting criteria of what science believes autism to be. It's that ever-shifting nature of the Western criteria that have bothered Chinese psychiatrists. Chinese psychiatrists, who have expressed doubts with the constant updates and diagnosis-associated changes of DSM and the awkwardly translated ICD, prefer the culturally appropriate Chinese Classification of Mental Disorders (CCMD-3) (Chen, 2002). There, though symptomatic diagnosis is largely standard, there are variances in interpretation and categorization between the CCMD and the DSM. For example, diagnosis of autism under CCMD-3 involves "interpersonal harm" with "qualitative damage" and "significantly impaired ability" in communication, as opposed to the "deficits" found in the DSM (Ming, 2012). Furthermore, thousands of years of cultural history have culminated in a socially accepted framework. This framework affects Chinese society's interpretation of autism. In framing autism, the five common themes found in the CCMD are:

> (1) As a basic life value, the Chinese stress a harmonious attitude toward nature; (2) Influenced by traditional medical concepts, the Chinese are concerned with balance and conservation for optimal health; (3) In their social organization, the Chinese value the family as the basic unit of life and resource for support; (4) The

Chinese emphasize social and interpersonal relations in
life situations; and (5) For coping with life situations, the
Chinese sanction practical and flexible adjustment.

(Ming, 2012)

It's important to bear in mind that the CCMD, flavored by
Traditional Chinese Medicine (TCM), largely views autism as a "yin"
disorder that manifests in social isolation, a lack of communication,
and apathy. It is thought that these symptoms are related
to underlying neurological aberrations; thus acupuncture is
thought to influence the regions of the brain associated with
autism (Clark and Zhou, 2005). Treatments for autism in China
begin with TCM. The more Western-style treatments, like applied
behavior analysis (ABA), are often disfavored or distrusted (Clark
and Zhou, 2005). Nevertheless, whether the diagnostic criteria
from ICD, the DSM, or the CCMD are used, the prevalence rates
of autism in China are about on par with those elsewhere in the
world (Wang et al., 2018).

It's that simple. Except… it's not.

What about the #actuallyautistic?

Several studies have found that a significant proportion (as much
as 40 percent) of individuals meeting the DSM-IV criteria for a
diagnosis of ASD did not meet the new criteria under the DSM-5
(Mazurek et al., 2017; Wing, Gould, and Gillberg, 2011; Worley and
Matson, 2012). The concerns raised by scholars and advocacy
groups about the clinical, research, and cultural implications of
those changes fell largely on unhearing ears. The most common
criticism of the DSM-5 definition of ASD is that the criteria were
too narrow and would result in excluding some individuals from

a diagnosis of autism and therefore exclude them from access to services they need (Carey, 2012). Those observations and warnings are now amplified with the even more restrictive DSM-5-TR. Nevertheless, the results of a lack of access to the process of diagnosis combined with more restrictive diagnostic criteria has led to the rapidly increasing phenomenon of self-diagnosis (Lewis, 2016). Many people now take online assessments and combine the results with their own lived experience to declare themselves to be autistic (de Broize et al., 2022).

In many Western cultures, the hashtag, #actuallyautistic, is used to self-identify oneself as autistic in social media spaces. Often, those using this label lack a formal diagnosis of autism (though some diagnosed autistics use this to declare allyship). Most who use the hashtag display with a great deal of pride (Gensic and Brunton, 2022). The problem for the self-diagnosed, however, is that they lack the force of law that the diagnosis gives them in achieving proper supports. They often note that the number of autistic people in each population is relatively stable over time, say 1:50. What changes is how society classifies autism (Zolyomi, Jones, and Kaftan, 2020). As the gatekeepers change their minds, the ratio has gone from 1:10,000 to 1:160 to 1:50. Now, will the DSM's Text Revision see that ratio trend back up toward the thousands again?

Structures and supports

As I have found at the many colleges that I have attended, schools will often do the minimum required to accommodate the disabled. They will often only grant access to help if a licensed professional writes a letter, sends it certified mail, and lists not only the diagnosis but the ways in which the disability impacts the student's educational experience. For me, my last school was so unhelpful that it took my medical team almost a semester to get the language right in their letter. Thus, what follows is a template that I created from that experience that can be used in requesting supports. It passed through one of the toughest gauntlets I've ever faced in attempting to receive help in accessing my teacher preparation training that was conducted online.

[Date of Letter]

To Whom It May Concern:

[Student name] (DOB: [student date of birth]) is currently under my psychiatric care for the following diagnosis which has been defined in the Diagnostic and Statistical Manual of Mental Disorders, 5th Edition, Text Revision (DSM-5-TR): Autism Spectrum Disorder (ASD).

[Student]'s diagnosis of ASD affects how language, oral and written, is used and understood, resulting in difficulty with making meaning of words in context. This impacts [insert appropriate pronoun] access to [in-person/virtual/asynchronous] instruction.

[Student]'s ASD diagnosis also affects [insert appropriate pronoun] ability to interact with related instructional tasks within the learning management system (LMS), which impacts [insert appropriate pronoun] involvement and progress in the curriculum.

To support [insert appropriate pronoun] learning, [student name] needs to use screen reading technology (text-to-speech) and browser plug-ins that process the text in a more accessible fashion. This requires all text in the LMS to be machine readable.

For live video presentations, [student] requires accurate captioning or subtitles for the video. For recorded video, [student] requires either captioning or a transcript of the presentation. For live in-person or virtual sessions, [student] requires an exemption from [name of school]'s policy against the recording of class sessions.

Please make these necessary accommodations to assist my patient in succeeding in [insert appropriate pronoun] educational goals.

[Signature]
[Provider's name and title]
[Date]

Notice that the doctor listed the diagnosis as well as how it impacts my involvement in a specific activity. This is no different than writing Impact of Disability Statements for Individualized Educational Plans. There, the format is simpler. One might look like the following:

Impact of Disability: [Student]'s eligibility of Autism Spectrum Disorder (ASD) affects [insert appropriate pronoun] ability to read related instructional tasks, decode, and comprehend grade level materials, which impacts [insert appropriate pronoun] involvement and progress in the general education curriculum in [subject].

The key to unraveling all this is being intentional. The care team must know the specific work or educational activity or environment that is impacted. They must know how to accommodate the needs of the student or employee. And they must phrase the request in a way that is acceptable to the company or school.

Here, I use work and school purposefully. Place is so important when considering autism and diagnoses. Under the current regime in most Western countries, if one neither works nor goes to school, a diagnosis of autism is rarely given. When it comes to autism and diagnosis, an individual is only disabled in relation to their ability to participate in some approved activity (e.g., work or school). Under the medical model, deficits become the focus of attention (Retief and Letšosa, 2018). If one is not participating in a societally approved function, such as work or school, is one disabled under the DSM/ICD definitions? The social model gets us part of the way toward an autistic identity. It can help with creating positive societal attitudes toward autistic people, shifting the burden of proving one's worth away from the autistic toward society (Woods, 2017).

Changing the conversation entirely, the Power Threat Meaning Framework (PTMF) examines the intersection of neoliberal values and increasingly scarce resources and opportunities for the disabled. Rather than require an autistic person to know what form to provide, or a care team to know which language is appropriate, the PTMF puts the burden on the employer or school. Under the PTMF, the following questions might be asked (Flynn and Polak, 2019):

- What brought a person to be diagnosed?
- When did they receive the diagnosis?
- Whose idea was it?
- What question was it hoped a diagnostic understanding would answer?
- How do referring services choose the people they refer for therapy or assessment?
- How are people streamed into specialist services from education and mental health systems as a whole?

Thus, under the PTMF, the system assumes that you're competent and that your identity is valid. It then seeks to know how best to support you.

What you need to know about requesting supports

If you are an adult, requesting supports from an employer can come with the risk of losing one's job. It may be that the work that you are doing cannot be accommodated in a way that is helpful to you (Madaus, 2008). I found this out during my time as a forensic scientist in police service. During that time, I was playing football in the National Public Safety Football League. One particularly tough game saw me injured. A very large defenseman decided to tackle the person with the ball by going through my knee. It took me over two years' intensive medical help to gain back about 80 percent functionality in my knee. But, when I could return to work on light duty, my unsympathetic supervisor took the occasion of my doctor's note to conduct what is known there as a "work fitness evaluation." Unfortunately for me, one of the requirements of my position was the ability to climb a ladder to a certain height with at least 50 lbs of gear. My note said that I was restricted from climbing and didn't list a date when this restriction would end. My pleas for sympathy went nowhere. My request for a reasonable accommodation fell upon the ears of an unreasonable person (Telwatte et al., 2017). In the end, I had to perform the test. I used my arms and my one good leg to get up and down the test ladder. It was incredibly painful, but I did it and kept my job. Had I not completed the task, I would have lost my career. Thus, be careful when asking for support.

If you are requesting accommodations from a school, they may not have the ability or desire to accommodate the student. I see this in my rural part of the world. Here, schools lack the funding to provide anything but the basic amount of support. The US Supreme Court decision in *Board of Education v. Rowley* (1982) found that "appropriate" does not mean "best." If a student's needs move beyond the school's ability to provide, the student may be bussed to a school that can help if the parents are willing to advocate for such a remedy. While this can be done at the school's expense or through a reimbursement to the family (FindLaw, 2016), here it means an almost two-hour one-way bus trip to get what the student requires. Having to catch a bus at 5:30am, knowing that the student will return around 6:00pm, puts an incredible strain on our local families.

What about the profoundly disabled?

We must return to the issue of functioning labels at this point. Remember, people change over time and in response to what's happening in different places. Nevertheless, there are some within the autistic community who won't. While I have moved from about a Level 2.5 to about a Level 1.5, others are born at Level 3 and stay there their whole life.

- Level 1: Requires Support.
- Level 2: Requires Substantial Support.
- Level 3: Requires Very Substantial Support.

I know families where their autistic loved one is profoundly disabled. Some have gained the ability to communicate thanks to grant-funded technological aids. Others have so terrorized their families who find themselves not knowing how to communicate even the most basic safety messages. From the sensory-seeking child who eats cat litter or runs after cars in the street, to the sensory-avoiding child who will melt down at the parent's attempt to put clothes on them, the life of a parent or caregiver of someone with such profound needs is one of the most stressful things imaginable. For these parents, ABA therapy is welcomed into their homes to help stop their kids from dangerous, even deadly, behaviors (Hoerricks, 2022).

One of the common conversations that happens among parents of profoundly disabled children centers around what will happen to their child when they are no longer able to provide for them (Ogston, Mackintosh, and Myers, 2011). More and more, we are seeing support groups feature legacy planning seminars and living trust workshops for families of autistic children.

(For a deeper dive into the WHO's International Classification of Functioning Disability and Health (ICF), a framework for investigating, assessing, and treating those with neurodevelopmental disorders holistically, see Bölte et al. (2021) at the end of this chapter.)

Let's debrief

As we've seen, the question of who is autistic is loaded with baggage. From an identity standpoint, one is autistic if one declares themself so. From a system standpoint, one is autistic only if one receives a diagnosis from an official agent of that system. That system, as we've seen, will change its mind occasionally as to what criteria are necessary to receive such a diagnosis.

Here's where you might get tripped up

You might be tempted, as I have been, to provide reasonable accommodations based upon a person's word that they need them. Lacking proof, you may choose simply to do the human thing, the kind thing. This may get you in trouble in some situations. Remember, if you are a teacher, you are an agent of that system and must play by its rules. For example, it may be easy to differentiate your instruction, but students without IEPs will not gain access to state-wide testing accommodations. Those are placed in the system by administrators based upon the designated supports listed in the IEP. If you are one of those administrators, will you open testing accommodations to all students? What would happen if you did?

On the other hand, being a loving and caring individual, you may refer the student for an evaluation. Hopefully, you've talked with the parent or guardian before doing so. Some parents do not want their children "in special ed." They reject that there's something "wrong" with their child and may thus refuse services. It's best to have good, regular communication with parents. In this way, you'll know when it might or might not be appropriate to bring up such topics.

Here's how we'll fix it

There is much that we can do to support autistic people in a variety of settings. Here's some examples of what that support can look like.

- Provide clear directions or instructions: it's important to provide autistic students or employees with clear, concise, and unambiguous directions or guidelines for performing their tasks. Thoroughly explain what's expected of them. Also make the effort to explain any unwritten rules. Given the prevalence of communications issues, it can be helpful to provide written instructions, syllabi, and so on, for autistic people so they have something to reference later when needed.

- Bring in outside support if you can: there are a variety of autism support services available for autistic people of all ages and their families. Many places have vocational or occupational services for disabled people that can make the process of finding and keeping a job much easier. These services often include providing on-site mentors and job coaches. Job coaches can provide additional support, such as securing transportation if the person doesn't drive.

• Provide reasonable accommodations: one of the best ways people can support autistic people is by providing reasonable accommodations. These include (but certainly aren't limited to) the following:

o Providing access to noise-reducing headphones.

o Turning off or dimming overhead lights.

o Avoiding direct eye contact. This often makes autistic people uncomfortable.

o Respecting personal space. Try using verbal praise to show kindness and appreciation instead of touch.

o Provide direction and instruction within small meetings. Avoid large groups and spaces as these can lead to sensory overload.

o Whenever possible, allow the individual to follow their own schedule to reduce their anxiety. With project-based exercises, you might be surprised at the methods the autistic person devises to accomplish the task. It may inform system-wide improvements in processes.

o Provide information about changes well in advance.

o Educate others about autism and how its strengths can benefit all.

o With the permission of both parties, designate a mentor or buddy.

In many cases, other people may not understand how to interact with autistic people. That's why education is so important. The person's colleagues should understand that there are genuine needs behind their reasonable accommodations. Training sessions (e.g., professional development) can help the entire team understand how to work together and deal with potential miscommunications. Consider creating a training document or series for your colleagues that explains what you've learned about autism. Open the room for people to discuss what they know and what they would like to know about autism. Build a collective understanding about what autism means within the spaces you inhabit.

Remember, it can be helpful for an autistic person to have a mentor or buddy that they can go to if they're anxious, confused, or stressed. This mentor should have some training in working with autistic people, so they know how to help and support their mentee.

Finally, provide consistent and constructive feedback. Consistent formative feedback is key to the improvement and success of any learner or worker. However, it's especially important for autistic people. Hold frequent, short meetings where you provide kind (but specific) feedback on how the individual is doing. When giving corrective feedback, it's important to thoroughly explain what the person is doing incorrectly, ensure they understand the problem, and direct them on how to improve. Provide a written plan if possible. Above all, highlight the person's knowledge and skill set and treat them as a valuable member of the group, just like any other member.

Now it's your turn

Considering what we've just covered, as well as the information from the previous chapters, create a brief narrative about the autistic person in a general sense. In between 1,500 and 2,000 words, describe how autism is viewed by the system as well as within the contexts in which you live and work. How does space/place influence who is considered to be autistic? Further, are the spaces you inhabit inclusive of autistic people or are there barriers to fully including them? If there are barriers, how would you engage in systems change leadership to remove these obstacles? Try to include a range of autistic people and places in your examples. Try also to include how you feel about what you've discovered as a part of your narrative.

Summary

In this chapter, we focused on the "who" of autism. We continued to dive into the autistic experience. Building upon the information about how autism is viewed around the world, we looked closer at how one is determined to be autistic. We became more familiar with diagnostic criteria used in making such determinations. We considered the question of who is autistic from multiple angles, that of the autistic person with a diagnosis, that of one without a diagnosis, that of the profoundly disabled, and those that care for the disabled. We saw, in our concluding activity, how much place can influence who is included in the autistic community. We can offer this new information and our insights to inform the larger conversation about how place, and one's relationship to place, can impact our experience of autism and the autistic identity.

Key vocabulary, terms, and people

- **Etymology.** The study of the origin of words and how words change over time.

- **Metaphysics.** The branch of philosophy that is concerned with the first principles of things, including concepts such as being, knowing, substance, cause, identity, time, and space.
- **Monogenesis.** The theory of human origins which posits a common descent for all human beings.
- **Polygenesis.** The theory of human origins which posits the view that the many human racial and cultural groups are of different origins. Historically, polygenism has been used to advance scientific racism and racial inequality.
- **Quality.** In philosophy, a quality is an attribute or a characteristic of an object.
- **Reasoning types.**

  o   Abductive reasoning: taking your best shot.
  o   Deductive reasoning: conclusion is guaranteed.
  o   Inductive reasoning: conclusion is merely likely.

- **Sublimination.** In chemistry, it describes what happens when a solid transforms directly into a gas. In psychology, Sigmund Freud used it to describe the transformation of the self to a higher level, or a transformation of "bad urges" into positive and productive activities. In practice, he used the term to describe a society civilizing or domesticating its people.
- **Louis Agassiz (1807–1873).** A Swiss-born American biologist and geologist. His prolific writings have often been used in support of scientific racism.
- **Edgar Rice Burroughs (1875–1950).** An American author best known for his adventure, science fiction, and fantasy books. He is known today as the creator of the characters Tarzan and John Carter. Burroughs either strategically placed

eugenics and scientific racism in his works or based his works entirely upon these themes.

- **Sigmund Freud (1856–1939).** An Austrian neurologist and psychoanalyst. His 1930 book, *Civilization and Its Discontents*, an examination of the tension between the individual and civilization, is one of the most influential and widely studied books in the modern field of psychology.
- **Emerson E. White (1829–1902).** An American educator, educational administrator, and author. As superintendent of Cincinnati's public schools, he decreased the reliance on written exams in favor of teacher recommendations as the basis for promoting students to the next grade level.

Building background knowledge

The following titles are not required reading but will serve those who study this topic by providing valuable context and background knowledge.

Aristotle and Sachs, J. (1999). *Aristotle's Metaphysics*. 2nd ed. Green Lion Press.

Bölte, S., Lawson, W. B., Marschik, P. B., and Girdler, S. (2021). Reconciling the seemingly irreconcilable: The WHO's ICF system integrates biological and psychosocial environmental determinants of autism and ADHD: The International Classification of Functioning (ICF) allows to model opposed biomedical and neurodiverse views of autism and ADHD within one framework. *BioEssays*, 43(9), 2000254.

Burroughs, E. R. (1917). *A Princess of Mars*. A. C. McClurg.

Cwik, J. C. and Margraf, J. (2017). Classification systems across the globe. In: S. Hofmann (ed.), *Clinical Psychology: A Global Perspective*. Wiley Blackwell, pp. 15–28.

Freud, S. (1930). *Das Unbehagen in der Kultur* [Civilization and Its Discontents]. Internationaler Psychoanalytischer Verlag.

Fromm, E. (1972). *Escape from Freedom*. Avon Books.

Schopler, E., Reichler, R. J., DeVellis, R. F., and Daly, K. (1980). Toward objective classification of childhood autism: Childhood Autism Rating Scale (CARS). *Journal of Autism and Developmental Disorders*, 10(1), pp. 91–103.

Vivanti, G., Hudry, K., Trembath, D., Barbaro, J., Richdale, A., and Dissanayake, C. (2013). Towards the DSM 5 criteria for autism: Clinical, cultural and research implications. *Australian Psychologist*, 48, pp. 258–261.

Volkmar, F. R. and Reichow, B. (2013). Autism in DSM-5: Progress and challenges. *Molecular Autism*, 4, p. 13.

White, E. E. (2013) [1886]. *The Elements of Pedagogy*. Book on Demand Ltd.

6
Why autism?

Learning objective

Students will be able to synthesize the intersecting identities within the autistic community.

Activity

Students research and report on the validity of diagnosis and self-diagnosis in various places in the world.

Introduction

Consider where we've been on our journey together. We've covered a tremendous amount of ground, yet have so far to go. We've saved the hardest question for last: **why**.

I think about all the places I've lived in as an autistic person. I think about my life before diagnosis as well as after. I think about the decades spent in therapy and the journey to my diagnosis. I think about all the prescriptions, potions, and notions offered by so-called medical experts. In all these situations, I was the outsider. I was the square peg. I was the one who needed fixing. I was the one who had to figure out how to fit into a world not designed with people like me in mind. In many spaces in which I interact today, sadly, this is still the case.

When we visited the legacy of the race scientists in previous chapters, we were horrified by the premise of eugenics – that there is one right way to be human and all other expressions should be extinguished from the planet. The eugenicists of the past sought to separate the acceptable from the unacceptable. History tells us what they did with those they considered "useless," but it's still hard to wrap our heads around the scope, scale, and premise of the killing regime. Like every conquering army before them, the race scientists decided who would live and who would not based upon expediency. They defined acceptable, and who would live, based upon their state's needs. They were the conquerors; the disabled and the different were the conquered. They just mindlessly destroyed millions of lives. Yet, as horrific as they were, they were no different than previous conquering regimes, such as the Spanish Conquistadores, the Mongol Hoard, and so on. Remember, never has a conquering army stopped to consider **why** the things they find are the way that they are. This effort has not abated. Today, it's the climate crisis and the resulting food insecurity that is driving these types of efforts. These experts cite the need to get to a sustainable population level using so-called one-child policies (Bradshaw and Brook, 2014). We have the benefit of history in this matter, that a large nation has already gone down this road and backed away once they realized the disaster that had resulted (Baochang et al., 2007). Yet at no time does anyone stop to consider that diversity within the human species is necessary and needed. We considered this question earlier and found that there were many times in humanity's past where the autistic neurotype was beneficial, perhaps instrumental in saving entire cultures from extinction.

In this sense, consider the opossum (*Didelphis virginiana*). It's not pretty, like a cat. It's not lovable, like a dog. You wouldn't want to keep it as a pet; they're quite nasty. Yet, it plays a valuable role in the ecosystem (Gardner, 1982). For some genetic reason, these omnivores require a lot of calcium in their diet. This causes them to seek out the old bones of dead animals to eat (McRuer and Jones, 2009). By doing this, they help clean up the environment, much in the same way as crows (Inger et al., 2016) and sharks (Fallows, Gallagher, and Hammerschlag, 2013) do. They help keep the lands of the Americas healthy. They're a vital part of the great food web. But so many people fear this little creature. People shoot it on sight. People go to great lengths to keep opossums off their property, likely without knowing why opossums exist. They simply react in fear and lash out (Animal Capture Wildlife Control, 2019).

My Tai Qi/Qi Gong master, Dr Yang, Jwing-Ming relates a story to illustrate this point – that of truly understanding something or someone (Yang, 2019b). He has said that he remembers the time when plastics were new to society. His White Crane master pulled an orange from his pocket and asked the assembled students to identify the object. All said, "orange." "No, it's not," was the master's reply. He then tossed the object to one of the students as he told the class that it was not an orange, but a plastic representation of an orange. He then pulled out a real orange and asked the students if the orange was sweet or sour. Of course, they couldn't tell from looking. So, he peeled it and divided it up. He gave each student a piece and asked the question again, now do you know this orange? The students gave their affirmative responses. He then stated to those assembled that they still do not **know** the orange. He told them that if they were really to **know** the orange, they would have to know about the conditions required to achieve such a quality of orange. The students had no idea how oranges are grown, so they were unable to respond with any useful information. He responded that looking is not as good as feeling, and feeling is still not good enough to be an expert. To be an expert in something, you must know how to create. You have to move beyond simply retelling or selling. To be an expert, your art or practice must be alive with deep feeling and authenticity. A similar explanation accompanies Dr Yang's (2019a) interpretation of the Dao De Jing, that when studying something so complex as Lao Zi's ancient treatise, one must have the same feeling and spiritual cultivation as the author. Now take these considerations and apply them to the research you've discovered on autism thus far. Do you see the same attempt at connection? Do you see deep feelings in these studies? Do you believe that the researchers had a deep and meaningful connection with those that they studied? I certainly haven't. To most, we're a curiosity; a problem to be solved.

Remember that medical science considers the autistic system to be a disordered neurotypical system (Lord et al., 2020). It seeks first to treat us with a variety of therapies while it works on a cure to ensure that what we now call autism never again is seen in the human genome (Hens, 2019). They do this without answering a basic question: why are autistic people still here after tens of thousands of years of evolution? If we were so undesirable and had no purpose in society, nature would have selected our genes out long ago (Reser, 2011). So, why are we autistics here?

When you examine the origin stories of the world's cultures, what do you find? What are the common themes (Sproul, 1979)? From the earliest records forward, we find in recorded mythology that humans were created by superior beings to serve various functions. The Sumerian deities wanted workers to mine gold and other precious materials (Stroe, 2020). In some cultures, such as the Norse, these creator deities wanted entertainment or companionship from their creation (Knutson, 2019). In still others, such as the Yorùbá (Bewaji, 2018) in Africa and the indigenous peoples of the Americas (Krueger, 2019), humanity serves as the caretakers of creation. In their mythology, humanity is a part of nature – coequal. We're not above it or separate from it. We certainly don't own it. As an interesting digression, when I dove deep into this topic in preparing for a bi-annual class on comparative philosophy that I teach each year, I found amazing similarities between the creation mythology of the Nde of the Sonoran Desert (US National Park Service, 2021) and Lurianic Kabbalah (DuQuette, 2001) – that the material world was "thought" into existence by the divine.

Justifying our existence

A rather vicious play in the eugenicists' playbook is the requirement that people justify their existence. If you search for the March 4th edition of London's *Daily Express* in 1910, you will find a speech given by Irish playwright and eugenicist George Bernard Shaw (Shaw, 1910). In it, he advocated for an "extensive use of the lethal chamber." Noting further that a "great many people would have to be put out of existence simply because it wastes other people's time to look after them." If you dig deeper into the internet, you will find a video of Shaw in a newsreel interview released on 5 March 1931 wherein he says the following:

> And I think it would be a good thing to make everybody come before a properly appointed board just as he might come before the income tax commissioners and say every five years or every seven years, just put them there, and say, sir or madam, now will you be kind enough to justify your existence? If you can't justify your existence; if you're not pulling your weight in the social boat; if you are not producing as much as you consume or perhaps a little more, then clearly we cannot use the big organization of our society for the purpose of keeping you alive, because your life does not benefit us, and it can't be of very much use to yourself.

Imagine that. Let that sit with you for a moment. Here, he's not just talking about the disabled. He's talking about everyone. Justify your existence… or else.

Now, take a moment and browse over to your favorite search engine. Type in "strengths of autistic people." Examine the results.

Regardless of your choice of tool, it's likely that the first few pages of results will be populated by pages seeking to quantify the autistic experience. It's been so bad that one study sought to quantify this phenomenon in a major US news outlet. The researchers predicted that the deficits view presented by the outlet would decrease over time as more positive narratives enter the conversation. Yet, their data showed this to not be the case; the deficits view did not change over time (Lewin and Akhtar, 2021). These reductive articles often feature stereotypes of autistic people in relation to their "worth" to society (Botha and Cage, 2022). In the world of curated search results, this is no accident. It's also quite a dangerous line of inquiry. Let's examine why.

More than 100 years ago, Francis Galton (1904) defined eugenics. He noted in *Eugenics: Its Definition, Scope, and Aims*, "[t]he aim of eugenics is to represent each class or sect by its best specimens; that done, to leave them to work out their common civilization in their own way" (Galton, 1904, p. 3). John Maynard Keynes, in *The End of Laissez-Faire* (1926), took the concept further, "[t]he time has already come when each country needs a considered national policy about what size of population, whether larger or smaller than at present or the same, is most expedient. And having settled this policy, we must take steps to carry it into operation. The time may arrive a little later when the community as a whole must pay attention to the innate quality as well as to the mere numbers of its future members."

Given what we've studied thus far, those quotes may no longer seem rather generic or esoteric. Yet, for an even more specific look at the early eugenics movement, we can turn to University of Reading researcher and author John S. Partington (2003) and his catalog of quotes in support of eugenics from the English author H. G. Wells. Here's just one of the viler of Wells' thoughts: "The way of nature has always been to slay the hindmost, and there is still no other way, unless we can prevent those who would become the hindmost being born. It is in the sterilization of failures, and not in the selection of successes for breeding, that the possibility of an improvement of the human stock lies" (Wells quoted in Galton, 1904, p. 11).

Eugenics as national health policy

As I write this, my county has been under the threat of yet another COVID-19 lockdown. A new variant is causing numbers of hospitalizations to climb once again. The health care system is under tremendous strain. The evening's news broadcast leads with an update about how many have died with COVID-19; with the prediction of more deaths to come unless we follow the ever-changing guidance from the Centers for Disease Control and Prevention.

The big urban cities in my country dominate the news cycles as more and more deaths are chalked up to the virus. Prediction models initially had the upper end of this pandemic at over 200,000 dead in America. Over the last month, that model has (thankfully) trended significantly lower.

Few countries have been spared from this medical crisis. In Western countries with national health systems, the discussion has turned to rationing care (Bhatia, 2020) and limiting "non-essential" visits to hospitals and clinics (Ahmed, Sanghvi, and Yeo, 2020). Many news stories featured a narrative that if a COVID patient goes into respiratory or cardiac arrest, the response team must take extra precautions and use protective equipment that's already in short supply (Binkley and Kemp, 2020). Otherwise, the experts tell us, doctors risk getting sick themselves or spreading the virus to other patients. Indeed, many health care professionals have been sickened by the virus. Some, sadly, have died (Ardebili et al., 2021).

Very few news outlets link eugenics, disabled people, and COVID-19 together in the same story. Yet, in the UK (Kavanagh et al., 2022) and in Italy (Faggioni, González-Melado, and Di Pietro, 2021), news reports illustrated the dilemma doctors faced as the disabled were seeking care. The systems were overwhelmed, and the official suggestion was that the disabled have a "do not resuscitate" order in place to save vital resources for those who really needed them (Taggart et al., 2022). Yes, hospitals were preparing guidelines on how to decide whose lives to prioritize if the health care system's resources are overwhelmed. Thankfully, these rationing policies and pandemic guidelines, which pose a grave threat to disabled people and those with chronic illnesses, were never fully implemented. But the mindset that led to the topic even being introduced remains.

Even today, with all the "awareness" campaigns, disabled people are seen by the system as less worthy of care, less valuable as human beings (Clifford and Dunk, 2021). If the system itself does not protect disabled people, some of us will pay the ultimate price at the hands of those who do not see our value.

Why would disabled patients be at risk?

At the heart of this problem lies eugenics and the quantification of the autistic experience. As the research clearly shows, the mindset behind eugenics has successfully informed the world's medical systems such that in a crisis, the disabled and the differently abled will not be chosen for heroic methods to save their lives (Botha and Cage, 2022).

Why? The world has been conditioned to believe that we're a drain on society since at least the time of George Bernard Shaw.

The news reports tell me, an autistic person, that the sum of my symptoms (as seen by society) add up to a net negative. Thus, I'm not worthy of the potential risk associated with resuscitating. This is the message autistic people are currently receiving via the evening news. Why would this be?

Consider the guidance given to new parents of autistic children by many support organizations (Chen et al., 2021). Better yet, we'll consider this topic from the point of view of my own parents. Rather than the typical "congratulations, ma'am," we now have the tragedy narrative – "I'm sorry ma'am, it's autistic." This would be followed up with the typical brochure describing all the ways in which our lives will be difficult, and our difficult lives will cause stress for our families and care providers (Factor et al., 2019).

- They'll likely have a hard time motivating themselves to stay on task and a difficulty in focusing on something other than their own interests (Jaswal and Akhtar, 2019).
- They'll have trouble following unwritten social rules. This can be helped through intensive therapy (Leaf et al., 2022). We'll give you brochures on that later.
- They'll likely miss the big picture (Jones, 2021).
- They'll have trouble with summarizing information to include in speech (Fennell and Johnson, 2022).
- They'll have difficulty with the generalization of concepts (degli Espinosa, 2022).
- They'll probably have an unbalanced set of skills (Kelly, O'Malley, and Antonijevic, 2018).
- They'll have trouble expressing their feelings in a way that other people would understand or expect (Kelly, O'Malley, and Antonijevic, 2018).

- They'll have trouble with basic functioning; hence they'll have difficulties in planning long-term activities (Stark and Lindo, 2022).
- You'll have trouble bonding with your child because people with autism have difficulty perceiving emotions of other people (Oakley et al., 2022).

As shocking as the above narrative is to read, it's paraphrased from a guide from a major US autism support agency. This is what a multi-million dollar "autism support" organization thinks of me. The linked research is provided in some of the cases to illustrate the underlying thought behind the statement. In other cases, the research directly refutes the statement and provides hope and guidance for autistic people.

Nevertheless, taking the opposing view, might there be a benefit to society for a group of people who are direct in their communication? Is there value to "matter of factness?" Is honesty of any value? Can we find worth in punctuality? What about loyalty? Considering what society calls our fixation on our particular special interests, what value could there be in a significant population of subject-matter experts within a society?

Circling back to the eugenics movement, let's again visit George Bernard Shaw (1931) and hear him again, in his own words, ask you and me to justify our existence. On the balance sheet of your life, do your strengths outweigh your challenges such that your life is a net benefit to society? How would a particular point sample, a day in your life chosen at random every five to seven years, compare to a normal distribution of the entirety of your life's experiences?

Speaking only for myself, I will say that the first 30 years of my life were quite a challenge; even more so given that there were no diagnoses or supports for the many things that place me firmly within the autism spectrum. If Shaw were to examine those years, he would likely conclude that I'm not worth the effort of being kept alive. Yet, my research has shown that the neurodivergent take a while to grow into the knowledge of how to operate our amazingly complex brains and bodies (Hoerricks, 2018).

But by way of example (accepting the premise that I must justify my autistic existence), since age 30 I've developed and practiced my use of the English language (my second, foreign language). As a non-verbal person, this takes time. Now that I have developed and practiced this skill, I've merged my interests into a single focus – working within, writing about, and teaching the many domains within the digital multimedia forensic sciences (a discipline that didn't exist when I was a child).

I think my experience speaks truth to Jared Reser's (2011) hypothesis, that what we now call autism has been with humanity for tens of thousands of years; that it's survived in our species through natural selection precisely because what makes us autistic has been useful to humanity's success as a species; and that autistic people have often been responsible for the very survival of our collective way of life.

You see, unlike the guidance noted above, as we've worked through this book together, we have seen that the neurodivergent generally have no problem perceiving the emotions of other people. We have discovered that the opposite is true. We found that many of us are highly empathic and get quickly overwhelmed by other people's uncontrolled emotions, especially when our empathy is combined with alexithymia. The inconvenient meltdowns and shutdowns are the inevitable result of our interactions with groups of neurotypicals who often have no concept or control of their own energies. Thus, many of us seek a sort of semi-isolation. During the COVID crisis, with its social distancing dictates, we're perfectly suited to ride it out. This is a social rule that we were already following.

With all of this in mind, we must get away from weighing people with a balance sheet. To paraphrase the founding documents of the US, we are all endowed by our Creator with certain inalienable rights, as well as strengths and weaknesses. The abled, the disabled, and the differently abled all have the same rights to life, liberty, and the possession of property. As philosopher Hannah Arendt noted famously, these rights do not end at arbitrary national or state borders. We each have these rights simply by being human (Arendt, 1970). We each do not need to justify ourselves to anyone; nor do we have to justify our right to exist.

Why autism then?

Consider the Danish philosopher, Søren Kierkegaard's idea that having consciousness of "self" is what separates humans from other animals. Yet, according to Kierkegaard, few humans make full use of this uniquely human capability. He observed that instead of making conscious decisions about how they want to live their lives, people simply follow convention. According to Kierkegaard, to have a meaningful life humans need to be able to choose and to act (Stack, 1973). When weighing the neurotypical and the neurodivergent considering Kierkegaard's existentialism, who is found living closer to their desires? If one of the complaints against the autistic neurotype is that we're too rigid, that once we've decided it's hard to get us to change, it sounds to me that we've made a conscious decision about how to live our lives; we don't want to follow convention for convention's sake. With that in mind, perhaps one of the reasons why autism exists is to remind humanity of what it means to live fully in the knowledge of "self."

Let's explore knowledge of self

Consider your intersectional identities. How many are biological? How many are related to place? How many are conscious choices or affiliations? How many are fluid or changeable?

My autistic identity is certainly based upon biology. My skin, hair, and eye color are based upon my northern European heritage. While they don't constitute an integral part of my identity, I recognize that the external features of my very tall body (my **conveyance**, as I call it) affect people's impressions of me. I had no choice of **conveyance** at birth. Mine came with an autistic operating system. Given my **conveyance**, I will not fit in in most places. They're simply not designed with people like me in mind.

When faced with not fitting in, many autistic people mask (Sedgewick, Hull, and Ellis, 2021). When we do, we approximate the behaviors we think the situation calls for, for better or worse. It takes a great deal of practice and effort to pull the act off to pass for neurotypical. Masking drains the person both physically and emotionally and often leads to meltdowns (Miller, Rees, and Pearson, 2021). Thus, finding the right place to live authentically becomes extremely important for autistic mental and physical health. For me, my place is under the dark skies of the rural mountains north of Los Angeles. It's quiet, remote, and secluded. Here, I can recharge. It coincidentally happens to be a place with a disproportionately high population of neurodivergent people.

As for gender and sexuality, you'll find that quite a few autistic people identify within the LGBTQ+ community (Moore et al., 2022). You'll also find that alexithymic autistic people often identify as demisexual (Lewis et al., 2021). For those of us that are alexithymic, that emotional/psychic connection that is possible with our hyper-empathic autistic system means that attraction is energy based, not necessarily based upon the other's **conveyance**. For me, growing up without an owner's manual for my system and lacking knowledge of "self," I was left wondering why I felt attracted to those who caught my fancy. The labels of Gay or Bi never felt quite appropriate for me. They were based, in my view, upon an attraction to or preference for the configuration of the conveyance. I understand now that my attractions are all energy based. It wasn't until recently that a term came along that captured the why of this aspect of my identity. I could now look back to high school with an explanation of why I felt a certain way about certain people. I wasn't fluid or changeable in this aspect. The language finally caught up with me and my experiences.

So, again, consider your intersectional identities. Dive deep into the **why** of the way in which you are. In your work with others, encourage them to do the same.

An evolutionary look

We learn in our Western schools that human life began in Africa a long time ago and spread out over the world. We also learn of a few near-extinction events that have happened that have caused the human population to get very small. For example, about 70,000 years ago, a massive eruption occurred in what is now Sumatra. That eruption coincided with a population constriction that is often cited as the cause of the relatively low genetic diversity across our species. Archaeological and genetic research suggests that as few as 2,000 humans were left alive by the eruption and its after-effects (Hancock, 2009). Moving forward from that chokepoint, humans have evolved a great deal of diversity. Why have these genetic adaptations come about? I know that I have light skin and eyes as a genetic gift from my ancestors. But why did these attributes evolve? What function do they serve? I have also been gifted my autistic system by those same forebears. Why did autism evolve not only among my ancestors, but everywhere on the planet? That autism tends to present in a similar fashion regardless of place or culture suggests a common genetic ancestor. Why then, after all these years of natural selection, is the autistic neurotype still among us if it has no use?

Again, why autism?

Remember that the American Psychiatric Association defines autism as having deficits in social communication and social interaction across multiple contexts as well as restricted, repetitive patterns of behavior, interests, or activities. Thus, in searching for the **why** of autism, we must consider why these aspects that are seen as deficits by the current medical establishment might be beneficial to our species. The Solitary Forager Hypothesis accounts for this in noting that many of the behavioral and cognitive tendencies that autistic individuals exhibit are viewed here as adaptations that would have complemented a solitary lifestyle (Reser, 2011).

It's important to note that all human behavioral and cognitive tendencies exist on a spectrum. We don't typically attach severity levels to neurotypical behaviors and traits. We simply note, for example, that there are extremely nice people and some that are not very nice. We see extremes in all groups, not just autistics.

Now let's break down those diagnostic features and see if we can find research that looks to answer our **why** questions. For example, **why** would deficits in social communication have an evolutionary advantage?

Setting up our graphic organizer

We can set up a graphic organizer to help us keep track of what we may find. The first row should contain the study's citation information. Then, I would create a column for each of the listed criteria from group A of DSM. Remembering that DSM-5-TR updates the language for group B to all the listed criteria, I would also set up columns for each of the group B criteria. We should also include a column to indicate if the study explicitly views autism as a positive factor in the studied population's lives. In other words, is the study set up to "treat" the observed behavior, or does the study attempt to quantify how the trait is beneficial and thus how it can be supported or encouraged. You will populate the rows with the information that you find.

A word of caution

Here's three things you should consider as you undertake this study. First, as you can already predict, there will be far more studies that look to "treat" us than look to quantify the ways in which our traits benefit society. Thus, the first several pages of results will return what the algorithm thinks you're looking for, such as treatments. You may end up 10 or 20 pages deep into the search results before finding your first significant study. Second, understanding that eugenic thought still holds a significant place in Western academic culture, your search may move beyond the English language. Google's translation service can help translate your search queries to return results in languages other than English. In doing so, you may find that autism is studied from unique angles far away from where you are today. Recall the example of Israel's military working out ways to integrate autistic people and their strengths into the defense of their nation. Studies and reports on that effort may be in Hebrew. Yes, Google Scholar does have settings that permit your English language searches to be returned in a few select languages. But if you limit yourself to just those select languages, you will necessarily miss results from India written in Hindi. Hindi is not a selection of the search>languages feature. If you choose to use this feature, click on the "hamburger icon" in the top left of the page. This will open the options. Click on Settings. Click on Languages. From there, you can choose how Google Scholar behaves. Notice that Hindi is not present. I tend to focus my searches in this way because, again, the algorithm is biased toward Western sources. When I want to find papers from a specific country, I will limit my search to that country's dominant language. Finally, Google Scholar isn't the only search engine out there. It is free, but it has its limitations. Your school's library may have paid for journal access, which will allow for a more comprehensive search and more meaningful results.

Some helpful search terms

From my own research efforts, I've accumulated a few search phrases in English and their counterparts in other popular languages. I'll share them with you here.

- When I want to find Chinese information on the benefits of social interaction deficits in autism, I will use the traditional Chinese phrase: 自閉症社交互動缺陷的好處. When the results are returned, my Chrome browser allows me to switch to English. I can then sift through the titles to find articles of interest. Once found, I can lift paragraphs from the papers and place them into Google Translate.

- When I want to find information on the benefits of social interaction deficits in autism from India, I will use the Hindi phrase: आत्मकेंद्रित में सामाजिक संपर्क घाटे के लाभ. Here I find that Chrome does not have a language adjustment. There aren't that many results returned, so my quick translation solution won't take up too much time.

- If I choose to look for results in German, I will use the phrase: Vorteile sozialer Interaktionsdefizite bei Autismus. Doing so yields many results, including a promising book by Georg Theunissen titled *Menschen im Autismus-Spektrum: verstehen, annehmen, unterstützen*, which translates as "People on the Autism Spectrum: Understand, Accept, Support."

You can repeat this exercise for each of the diagnostic criteria and behaviors. Be sure to search for benefits, not just treatments. In the end, you should have a comprehensive and current view on the current state of the research. From there, you can postulate the **why** based upon your results.

Debrief

As you went through the exercise, you likely noticed trends in the search results. For example, I found about a third as many results in Chinese as I did in German. Was this due to an algorithmic bias toward the DSM in searches performed in the West? Did the algorithm disfavor CCMD-based results? Unfortunately, we can't know. Continuing, I hardly found any autism scholarship published in Hindi. What I did find written in Hindi was information from support groups that generally referred to studies from the US and western Europe, which were all written in English. If you're an Indian parent looking into the efficacy of treatments that have been recommended for your child, and you don't read academic English, you may not be able to effectively use the information that you find.

You may also have found that how autism is viewed within a culture will influence how it is studied, and for what purpose. For example, the focus of most American and Chinese research focuses on how to mitigate autistic behaviors such that students can attend regular schools and access the general education curriculum, which will lead to their having productive lives. In Germany, the focus seems to be on how to integrate the so-called high-functioning autistic adults into the workforce. Less time is spent considering the integration of the profoundly disabled or their quality of life.

When performing searches such as this, I must remind myself of Dr Yang's advice on learning. I try to empathize with the other culture, get to know them more than superficially. This helps me to better interpret the results.

Here's where you might get tripped up

Unfortunately, depending on where you are in the world, certain scholarship might be unavailable. As I write this book, the US is picking a fight with both China and Russia. Both are significant sources of scholarship on autism. In response to my government's call to action, many universities have closed access to Russian institutions and journals. China may soon be next. These unfortunate obstacles can't be easily or safely overcome.

Here's how we'll fix it

Researchers have long used social media apps to communicate with their counterparts around the globe. Although Facebook and Twitter claim a global reach, their content is often blocked by internal censors in many countries. Thus, you'll want to gain familiarity with their analogues in the countries in which you wish to conduct your research. For example, many people in Russia use either VK.com or OK.ru. In China, you may find researchers using Weibo's microblogging feature. Registering with Weibo as a foreign citizen is easy.

Now it's your turn

Consider what we've just covered about how different cultures may view autism. You may have found it difficult to find research on autism showing it to be a net benefit to society. For our concluding activity, we'll use the skills we've just practiced to turn our attention to a separate but equally significant question: given the changes to the DSM, what are a particular culture's views on the validity of autism diagnoses, including self-diagnosis? Many young undiagnosed autistic people believe that a diagnosis will convince those around them to take their needs seriously (McDonald, 2020). They often fail to understand that someone who doesn't respect you and your needs isn't likely to change when presented with a piece of paper. These attitudes are present in a variety of contexts. Here, make it personal. Study your place and context. See what information is available. Construct a graphic organizer or add to what you've worked on in this chapter to collect your information. Afterward, create a brief narrative about what you discovered (1,500–2,000 words). Does your "place" lean into the strengths and benefits of autistic people? Do they view autistic people, even or especially the self-diagnosed, as valid and honor their requests for support and inclusion? Try to include how you feel about what you've discovered as a part of your narrative.

Summary

In this chapter, we focused on the **why** of autism. We dove deep into the autistic experience. We were faced with some obstacles to conducting research. We became familiar with some tools and techniques to help us in our inquiries. Continuing in the realization that not enough has been written and collected about the benefits autistic people bring to our communities, we assembled data and a narrative of our culture's view of autism. We can offer our new information and insights to inform the larger conversation about how place, and one's relationship to place, can impact our experience of autism and autistic identity.

Key vocabulary, terms, and people

- **Dunn's Four Quadrant Model of Sensory Processing.** Occupational therapist Winnie Dunn built upon the work of Jean Ayres and created a model based on two constructs: one's neurological thresholds and the resulting behavioral response.

- **Existentialism.** A western European philosophical interpretation of humanity's existence in the world that concentrates upon life's concreteness as well as its challenging nature. At its core, it is the investigation of the meaning of Being.

- **Masking.** Autistic masking, camouflaging, or compensating is a conscious or unconscious withholding of natural behavioral responses. It is a hiding, minimizing, modifying, or controlling of the behaviors typically associated with the autism neurotype. It has been likened to improvisational acting and is linked to an autistic person's attempts to fit into a particular environment that has not been designed with autistic people in mind. It is most common in social/workplace situations where autistic people mix with neurotypical people.

- **Sensory-avoiding behavior.** Sensory-avoiding behavior is a term used to describe a large class of behaviors that are used manage one's hypersensitivity. Most sensory avoiders are oversensitive and experience sensory inputs more intensely than the average person. Thus, they tend to avoid many sensory inputs as they are overwhelming.

- **Sensory-seeking behavior.** Sensory-seeking behavior is a term used to describe a large class of behaviors that are used to meet a sensory need. Individuals engage in sensory seeking to obtain feedback from the environment. No two sensory-seeking people demonstrate the same seeking behaviors.

- **A. Jean Ayres, PhD, OTR (1920–1988).** An American occupational therapist and educational psychologist. She developed, practiced, and tested a theory of sensory integration, which she believed to be fundamental to people's ability to be successful in daily life activities. She developed tests of various aspects of sensory integration and invented the equipment that is used in the practice.

- **Marjorie Glicksman Grene (1910–2009).** An American philosopher. She was one of the first philosophers to question the synthetic theory of evolution, which combines Darwin's theory of evolution, Mendel's understanding of genetic inheritance, and the more recent discoveries by molecular biologists. Woven through her many works is a common question about the qualities that "make" a person, noting that people become themselves by the way they participate in their culture.

- **Watsuji Tetsurō (1899–1960).** A Japanese philosopher and historian. Credited with the introduction of existentialism into Japan, Tetsurō emphasized the human being as both an individual entity as well as a social being who is integral to, or interdependent with, society.

Building background knowledge

The following titles are not required reading but will serve those who study this topic by providing valuable context and background knowledge.

DuQuette, L. M. (2001). *The Chicken Qabalah of Rabbi Lamed Ben Clifford: Dilettante's Guide to What You Do and Do Not Need to Know to Become a Qabalist*. Weiser Books.

La Rowe, K. (2005). *Breath of Relief: Transforming Compassion Fatigue into Flow (with DVD)*. Acanthus Publishing.

Le Guin, U. K. (2019). *Lao Tzu: Tao Te Ching: A Book about the Way and the Power of the Way*. Reissue ed. Shambhala.

Sproul, B. (1979). *Primal Myths: Creation Myths Around the World*. HarperOne.

Vasiliev, V. (2006). *Let Every Breath... Secrets of the Russian Breath Masters*. Russian Martial Art.

Yang, J. M. (2019a). *The Dao De Jing: A Qigong Interpretation*. 1st ed. YMAA Publication Center.

Yang, J. M. (2019b). *The Dao in Action: Inspired Tales for Life*. 1st ed. YMAA Publication Center.

7
Summary

Review

In the preceding chapters, we have attempted to achieve a grand goal. We set out to not only frame autism but also to frame the ideal situation and conditions whereby autistic people could thrive. To complete this goal, I did not dictate these terms from my point of view or context but rather provided a framework for learners to discover these for themselves. Because autism is present in all cultures and places, and the experience of being autistic in a certain place varies according to culture and place, I hoped that in structuring the book in the way that I have, we could piece together a coherent whole from the experiences and records of those using this book to aid in their discoveries.

In Chapter 1, I presented my unique lived experience of being a non-verbal autistic person across five decades of living and working across three continents. In doing so, identity and its intersectional impact were shown as fluid as place and time changed. The narrative was not provided to cement an autistic way of being modeled upon my life, but to provide a glimpse of how the view of autism has evolved over time. With sharing my experiences of living under the regimes of the several modern revisions of the DSM, it was hoped that the learner could envision the impact on autistic lives as distant experts refine their view of autism over time.

In Chapter 2, I asked, "what is autism?" There, the learner was introduced to Reser's Solitary Forager Hypothesis of Autism. We worked from the premise that the autistic system is the result of tens of thousands, if not hundreds of thousands, of years of natural selection. With natural selection in mind, I posited that the autistic system works as designed, and then we unpacked the design to uncover where and when it might have been advantageous to have autistic people among a population.

In Chapter 3, I asked, "when is autism?" There, I hoped to discover when autism first appeared in the human genetic record. Once determined, we worked forward in time to explore the many times and places in which autism may have been instrumental in the preservation of humanity. We explored various contexts, and I asked learners to dive deep into their own cultural past, or the past of another culture of their choosing, to discover a time and place where the autistic neurotype might have been instrumental in saving a society from destruction or extinction. In doing so, we discovered how the autistic neurotype was an essential part of human diversity. Along the way, learners were introduced to the horrors of scientific racism, as well as to Dr Sukhareva, who accurately described what we now call autism decades before the scientific racists of the West.

In Chapter 4, I asked, "where is autism?" Having gained the understanding that autism is present in all cultures, across time, and across the gender spectrum, we further explored how the experience of autism can vary from place to place. Here, we found that not all cultures are welcoming of autistic people. This lack of acceptance was demonstrated within several research papers and informational websites. In these places, autistics and their advocates face an uphill, sometimes violent, climb to full inclusion and integration within society. Learners were provided with a method of finding and organizing research on autism within their local contexts.

In Chapter 5, I asked, "who is autistic?" Given the changing criteria for diagnosing autism in the Western world, we explored how place influences access to diagnosis, a vital piece of the autistic identity. We then moved beyond the West to discover how people of other cultures identify and include (or exclude) the autistic people who inhabit their place. There, I shared insights on the power of determining one's own identity, and the importance of being in control of it. The models of disability were further explored with the hope of discovering a proper framing for autistic identity. Here, we saw how self-diagnosis may be facilitated and how it may impact one's identity in each place.

In Chapter 6, I asked, "why autism?" We continued the exploration of diagnosis and self-diagnosis, wondering why someone would choose to be a part of a community that is often on the margins of society. We wondered further at the benefit of self-diagnosis and why it has become more popular in Western societies. We investigated the influence of place on access to diagnosis and diagnostic prevalence. This chapter took the process of discovery in a more philosophical direction, unpacking the autistic neurotype in terms of the ancient philosophical systems of the world and their ideas as to why the varied species and varieties of species are here on this planet. We explored the potential perils of revealing one's diagnosis in a world with scarce medical resources. We uncovered potential bias in the research around autism and found that the influence of scientific racism was still a factor. Despite it all, we found hope in the greater representation of autistic researchers in conducting research on autism.

A cohesive view of autism

In Chapter 6, we examined common statements on autistic traits found in the brochures of the many autism support organizations that serve our community. We attached relevant research to show that either the statements were false or biased. In Chapter 5, we explored the power of name and how or why names are chosen. These two chapters can inform the creation of a cohesive view of autism. This cohesive view necessarily requires that the autistic people, the neurodivergent, decide for themselves not only the name of their identity and neurotype, but on what terms they will interact within a culture.

From this standpoint, autism as "selfism" can be seen as the dominant culture's comment on the person's position relative to society – that of not caring or wanting to be a part of it. We can ask if one who possesses this neurotype would wish to be viewed in this way. Pushing back on this narrative, some in the community have published papers and books to carve out space and control the narrative from an authentic perspective. In one such book (Walker, 2021), the author lists several definitions that have been accepted by a large part of the neurodivergent community. There, neurodivergent means having a system that functions in ways which diverge significantly from the dominant societal standards of "normal." From there, the author defines neurodiversity as the diversity of all human minds, or the infinite variation in neurocognitive functioning within humanity. To get there, the author presents a paradigm of neurodiversity. The neurodiversity paradigm is a specific perspective on neurodiversity that sees neurodiversity as a natural, normal, and valuable form of human diversity; that the idea that there is one "normal" or "healthy" type of brain or mind, or one "right" style of neurocognitive functioning (as we saw with scientific racism), is a culturally constructed fiction that is lacking in validity; and that the social dynamics that manifest regarding neurodiversity are similar to the social dynamics that manifest in regard to the other forms of human diversity.

Attempting to trace the roots of this phenomenon, that of the dominant culture naming and claiming that which it surveys, another author posits (Kahn, 2022) that colonialism hasn't disappeared into the background of history. She sees capitalism as modern colonialism, and recoils at its attempt to enforce unnatural hierarchies within societies in its constant pursuit of profits. Perhaps, given Kierkegaard's notion of the knowledge of self, and Chapter 6's exploration of the neurodivergent being more knowledgeable and less willing to compromise as regards self, the colonial mindset sees the neurodivergent as needing to be brought to heel, to conform, and to fit within its profit-driven schemes. This is a possible source of the seeming need for cures and therapies.

Given all that we've learned about autism and neurodivergence, and that which we are still discovering, is the pursuit of a genetic fix for neurodivergence ethical? If you are autistic, would you accept an injectable therapeutic that promised to rewrite your genetic code to make you "normal" (Moon, 2002)? What if one was available, but you rejected it? How do you think society, or your family, would view your choice? What if society gave you no choice in the matter?

Taking a step back, what if we simply reframe what we know about autism? What the DSM calls Autism Spectrum Disorder (ASD) is simply a developmental difference rooted in the human genome. Autistic people may behave, communicate, interact, and learn in ways that are both similar and different from those around them. Like all humans, the abilities of autistic people can vary significantly relative to task, time, and/or place. For example, some autistic people may have advanced conversation skills, while others may be non-verbal. Some non-verbal people can learn to use the dominant language of their culture over time, others cannot. Some autistic people need a lot of help in their daily lives; others can work and live with little to no support. Seen in this way, autism is no different than any other part of the human condition. We are born needing the support of our mother to survive. We grow up and into our abilities, eventually separating from our care providers to a more independent life. Toward the end, our bodies again require support to function. The severities of each stage depend upon individual and cultural circumstances.

Final thoughts

As your author and guide, it is my sincere hope that you have found value in this experience. Through the exercises, you have collected valuable data and knowledge. Please do not hide what you've found; rather share it with the world. If you see something working, call the world's attention to it. If you see injustice, like that we found in Myanmar, name it and call it out for what it is. If you have engaged with this work because you work with autistic people and seek to know more about autism, don't stop here. Keep going in your inquiry. Remember, if you've met one autistic person, you've met one autistic person… once. If you knew me in high school, for example, you would not think me capable of producing such a work as this today. Yet here we are.

I must name and acknowledge the enormous privilege that I have in being able to share this work with you. I understand that my place in this world affords me the freedom to do so, and that other places and contexts force autistic people and their families into the margins. It is my sincere hope that humanity shifts its trajectory away from the scientific racists and ableists toward a more just and equitable path, one where differences are celebrated and accommodated. Hopefully, with your help, we can create the change we seek.

References

Chapter 1

Armstrong, P. (2022). Bloom's Taxonomy. [Online] Vanderbilt University Center for Teaching. Available at: https://cft.vanderbilt. edu/guides-sub-pages/blooms-taxonomy (accessed 14 August 2022).

Autistic Bride. (2019). Autism Parents™ vs. parents of autistics. [Online] Available at: http://autisticbride.co.uk/2019/07/22/aut ism-parents-vs-parents-of-autistics

British Broadcasting Corporation (BBC). (2020). Coronavirus: Autistic support group "told it needed DNR orders." [Online] Available at: www.bbc.com/news/uk-england-somerset-52217 868 (accessed 13 August 2022).

Campisi, L., Imran, N., Nazeer, A., Skokauskas, N., and Azeem, M. W. (2018). Autism spectrum disorder. *British Medical Bulletin*, 127(1), pp. 91–100.

Gernsbacher, M. A. and Yergeau, M. (2019). Empirical failures of the claim that autistic people lack a theory of mind. *Archives of Scientific Psychology*, 7(1), pp. 102–118.

Hoerricks, J. (2022). Are there two sides to the ABA coin? The AutSide. [Online] Available at: https://autside.substack.com/p/ are-there-two-sides-to-the-aba-coin

Lord, C., Brugha, T. S., Charman, T., Cusack, J., Dumas, G., Frazier, T., Jones, E. J., Jones, R. M., Pickles, A., State, M. W., and Taylor, J. L. (2020). Autism spectrum disorder. *Nature Reviews Disease Primers*, 6(1), pp. 1–23.

Lord, C., Elsabbagh, M., Baird, G., and Veenstra-Vanderweele, J. (2018). Autism spectrum disorder. *The Lancet*, 392(10146), pp. 508–520.

Millman, C. (2020). Why autism ABA goes against everything Skinner believed in. NeuroClastic. [Online] Available at: https://neuroclastic.com/why-autism-aba-goes-against-everything-b-f-skinner-believed-in (accessed 6 August 2022).

Opai, K. (2017). A time and space for takiwātanga. *Altogether Autism Journal*, 2, p. 13.

Reser, J. (2011). Conceptualizing the autism spectrum in terms of natural selection and behavioral ecology: The solitary forager hypothesis. *Evolutionary Psychology: An International Journal of Evolutionary Approaches to Psychology and Behavior*, 9(2), pp. 207–238.

Stenson, J. (2019). Why the focus of autism research is shifting away from searching for a "cure." NBC News. [Online] Available at: https://nbcnews.com/health/kids-health/cure-autism-not-so-fast-n1055921 (accessed 7 August 2022).

Zadrozny, B. (2019). Parents are poisoning their children with bleach to "cure" autism. These moms are trying to stop it. NBC News. [Online] Available at: https://nbcnews.com/tech/internet/moms-go-undercover-fight-fake-autism-cures-private-facebook-groups-n1007871 (accessed 7 August 2022).

Chapter 2

Botha, M., Hanlon, J., and Williams, G. L. (2021). Does language matter? Identity-first versus person-first language use in autism research: A response to Vivanti. *Journal of Autism and Developmental Disorders*. [Online] Available at: https://doi.org/10.1007/s10803-020-04858-w (accessed 6 August 2022).

Boucher, J. (2001). "Lost in a sea of time": Time-parsing and autism. In: C. Hoerl and T. McCormack, eds., *Time and Memory: Issues in Philosophy and Psychology*. Oxford University Press, pp. 111–135.

Bradley, J. (2013). Two visions for understanding illness: DSM and the International Classification of Diseases. The Conversation. [Online] Available at: https://theconversation.com/two-visions-for-understanding-illness-dsm-and-the-international-classificat ion-of-diseases-14167 (accessed 7 August 2022).

Callahan, M. (2018). "Autistic person" or "person with autism": Is there a right way to identify people? [Online] Available at: https://news.northeastern.edu/2018/07/12/unpacking-the-deb ate-over-person-first-vs-identity-first-language-in-the-autism-community (accessed 13 August 2022).

Cardoso-Martins, C. and Da Silva, J. R. (2010). Cognitive and language correlates of hyperlexia: Evidence from children with autism spectrum disorders. *Reading and Writing*, 23(2), pp. 129–145.

Centers for Disease Control and Prevention (CDC). (2022). Autism Spectrum Disorder. [Online] Available at: www.cdc.gov/ncbddd/ autism/hcp-dsm.html (accessed 13 August 2022).

Davies, J., Heasman, B., Livesey, A., Walker, A., Pellicano, E., and Remington, A. (2022). Autistic adults' views and experiences of requesting and receiving workplace adjustments in the UK. *PloS One*, 17(8), e0272420.

Fang, Y., Luo, J., Boele, M., Windhorst, D., van Grieken, A., and Raat, H. (2022). Parent, child, and situational factors associated with parenting stress: A systematic review. *European Child & Adolescent Psychiatry*, pp. 1–19.

Gernsbacher, M. A., Morson, E. M., and Grace, E. J. (2016). Language and speech in autism. *Annual Review of Linguistics*, 2, pp. 413–425.

Hus, V. and Lord, C. (2014). The Autism Diagnostic Observation Schedule, Module 4: Revised algorithm and standardized severity scores. *Journal of Autism and Developmental Disorders*, 44(8), 1996–2012.

Khan, A. (2022). Decolonizing= abolishing bioessentialism & the neurodivergent/neurotypical binary. [Online] Available at:

https://wokescientist.substack.com/p/decolonizing-abolishing-bioessentialism (accessed 13 September 2022).

Kim, S. A. (2022). Transition to kindergarten for children on the autism spectrum: Perspectives of Korean–American parents. *Journal of Autism and Developmental Disorders*, pp. 1–16.

Leekam, S. R., Libby, S. J., Wing, L., Gould, J., and Taylor, C. (2002). The Diagnostic Interview for Social and Communication Disorders: Algorithms for ICD-10 childhood autism and Wing and Gould autistic spectrum disorder. *Journal of Child Psychology and Psychiatry, and Allied Disciplines*, 43(3), pp. 327–342.

Lightner, L. (2022). Educational autism | What's the difference between a medical and a school diagnosis of autism? A Day in Our Shoes. [Online] Available at: https://adayinourshoes.com/autism-whats-the-difference-between-medical-and-educatio nal-diagnoses/#h-medical-vs-educational-diagnosis (accessed 6 August 2022).

Lord, C., Risi, S., DiLavore, P. S., Shulman, C., Thurm, A., and Pickles, A. (2006). Autism from 2 to 9 years of age. *Archives of General Psychiatry*, 63(6), pp. 694–701.

Marriott, E., Stacey, J., Hewitt, O. M., and Verkuijl, N. E. (2022). Parenting an autistic child: Experiences of parents with significant autistic traits. *Journal of Autism and Developmental Disorders*, 52(7), pp. 3182–3193.

Mumtaz, N., Fatima, T., and Saqulain, G. (2022). Perception of burden and stress among mothers of autistic children in Pakistani cultural background. *Iranian Rehabilitation Journal*, 20(1), pp. 43–52.

Nation, K., Clarke, P., Wright, B., and Williams, C. (2006). Patterns of reading ability in children with autism spectrum disorder. *Journal of Autism and Developmental Disorders*, 36(7), pp. 911–919.

Neely, L., Gerow, S., Rispoli, M., Lang, R., and Pullen, N. (2016). Treatment of echolalia in individuals with autism spectrum disorder: A systematic review. *Review Journal of Autism and Developmental Disorders*, 3(1), pp. 82–91.

Ono Academic College. (2022). Roim Rachok Program. [Online] Available at: www.roim-rachok.org/english (accessed 13 August 2022).

Ostrolenk, A., d'Arc, B. F., Jelenic, P., Samson, F., and Mottron, L. (2017). Hyperlexia: Systematic review, neurocognitive modelling, and outcome. *Neuroscience & Biobehavioral Reviews*, 79, pp. 134–149.

Prizant, B. M. (1983). Language acquisition and communicative behavior in autism: Toward an understanding of the "whole" of it. *Journal of Speech and Hearing Disorders*, 48(3), pp. 296–307.

Roberts, J. M. (2014). Echolalia and language development in children with autism. In: J. Arciuli and J. Brook (eds.), *Communication in Autism*. John Benjamins Publishing Company, pp. 55–74.

The Royal Children's Hospital Melbourne. (2022). Autism assessment ages 0–6. [Online] Available at: www.rch.org.au/ autism/autism_assessment/Autism_assessment_ages_0-6 (accessed 13 August 2022).

Rutter, M., LeCouteur, A., and Lord, C. (2003, 2008). Autism Diagnostic Interview–Revised. Los Angeles, CA: Western Psychological Services.

Sanz-Cervera, P., Pastor-Cerezuela, G., Fernández-Andrés, M. I., and Tárraga-Mínguez, R. (2015). Sensory processing in children with Autism Spectrum Disorder: Relationship with non-verbal IQ, autism severity and Attention Deficit/Hyperactivity Disorder symptomatology. *Research in Developmental Disabilities*, 45, pp. 188–201.

Seymour, L. (2022). Shakespearean echolalia: Autism and versification in *King John*. *Shakespeare*, 18(3), pp. 335–351.

Silvers, A. (2009). An essay on modeling: The social model of disability. In: D. C. Ralston and J. Ho (eds.), *Philosophical Reflections on Disability*. Springer, pp. 19–36.

Skuse, D., Warrington, R., Bishop, D., Chowdhury, U., Lau, J., Mandy, W., and Place, M. (2004). The Developmental, Dimensional, and Diagnostic Interview (3di): A novel computerized assessment for autism spectrum disorders. *Journal of the American Academy of Child and Adolescent Psychiatry*, 43(5), pp. 548–558.

Therapeutic Pathways. (2021). Who can diagnose autism? [Online] Available at: www.tpathways.org/faqs/who-can-diagnose-autism (accessed 13 August 2022).

Walker, N. (2022). Neurodiversity: Some basic terms and definitions. [Online] Available at: https://neuroqueer.com/neurodiversity-terms-and-definitions (accessed 14 August 2022).

Wen, B., van Rensburg, H., O'Neill, S., and Attwood, T. (2022). Autism in the Australian workplace: The employer perspective. *Asia Pacific Journal of Human Resources*. https://doi.org/10.1111/1744-7941.12333.

Woods, W. (2017). Exploring how the social model of disability can be re-invigorated for autism: In response to Jonathan Levitt. *Disability & Society*, 32(7), pp. 1090–1095.

World Health Organization. (2022). 6A02 Autism spectrum disorder. [Online] Available at: https://icd.who.int/browse11/l-m/en#/http://id.who.int/icd/entity/437815624 (accessed 6 August 2022).

Chapter 3

Abubakar, A., Ssewanyana, D., and Newton, C. R. (2016). A systematic review of research on autism spectrum disorders in sub-Saharan Africa. *Behavioural Neurology*. DOI: 10.1155/2016/3501910.

Applied Behavior Analysis Programs Guide. (2022). History's 30 most famous people with autism. [Online] Available at: www. appliedbehavioranalysisprograms.com/historys-30-most-inspir ing-people-on-the-autism-spectrum (accessed 7 August 2022).

Black, E. (2012). *War Against the Weak: Eugenics and America's Campaign to Create a Master Race*. Dialog Press.

Bohling, S., Croucher, K., and Buckberry, J. (2022). The bio-archaeology of disability: A population-scale approach to investigating disability, physical impairment, and care in archaeological communities. *International Journal of Paleopathology*, 38, pp. 76–94.

Cahill, T. (1996). *How the Irish Saved Civilization: The Untold Story of Ireland's Heroic Role from the Fall of Rome to the Rise of Medieval Europe*. Vol. 1. Anchor.

Cooper, K., Russell, A., Calley, S., Chen, H., Kramer, J., and Verplanken, B. (2022). Cognitive processes in autism: Repetitive thinking in autistic versus non-autistic adults. *Autism*, 26(4), pp. 849–858.

Dou, H. (2022). *Effects of Social Exclusion, Observational Learning, and Oxytocin on Fear Learning and Generalization: Evidence from Behavioral and Brain Activity Studies*. Doctoral dissertation. University of Jyväskylä (Finland), School of Education and Psychology.

Edwards, S. (2015). Nightmares and the brain. Harvard Medical School. [Online] Available at: https://hms.harvard.edu/news-eve nts/publications-archive/brain/nightmares-brain (accessed 6 August 2022).

Feinstein, A. (2011). *A History of Autism: Conversations with the Pioneers*. John Wiley & Sons.

Hammond, T. (2022). Tiffy's "big" book of ABA+ race, intersectionality, parenthood, and compliance. Buy Me a Coffee. [Online] Available at: www.buymeacoffee.com/fidgetsandfries/ e/84228 (accessed 25 August 2022).

Jackson, J. P., Weidman, N. M., and Rubin, G. (2005). The origins of scientific racism. *The Journal of Blacks in Higher Education*, 50(50), pp. 66–79.

Jogoleff, C. (2012). *Criminal Reproduction: Early Eugenics and Gendered Imprisonment in California*. UCLA: Center for the Study of Women. [Online] Available at: https://escholarship.org/uc/item/78f522b7 (accessed 13 August 2022).

Kirschenbaum, L. A. (2013). *Small Comrades: Revolutionizing Childhood in Soviet Russia, 1917–1932*. Routledge.

Kobenan, B. (2012). Autism Community of Africa. Autism Around the Globe. [Online] Available at: www.autismaroundt heglobe.org/story/autism-community-of-africa (accessed 7 August 2022).

Laughlin, H. H. (1922). *Eugenical Sterilization in the United States*. Psychopathic Laboratory of the Municipal Court of Chicago.

Lewis, L. F. (2017). A mixed methods study of barriers to formal diagnosis of autism spectrum disorder in adults. *Journal of Autism and Developmental Disorders*, 47(8), pp. 2410–2424.

Manouilenko, I. and Bejerot, S. (2015). Sukhareva—prior to Asperger and Kanner. *Nordic Journal of Psychiatry*, 69(6), pp. 1761–1764.

McLeod, S. A. (2012). What is the zone of proximal development? *Simply Psychology*. [Online] Available at: www.simplypsychology. org/Zone-of-Proximal-Development.html (accessed 13 August 2022).

Minkova, E. (2012). Pedology as a complex science devoted to the study of children in Russia: The history of its origin and elimination. *Psychological Thought*, 5(2), pp. 83–98.

Novin, A. and Meyers, E. (2017). Making sense of conflicting science information: Exploring bias in the search engine result page. In: R. Nordie, N. Pharo, L. Freund, B. Larsen, and D. Russel (eds.), *Proceedings of the 2017 Conference on Human Information*

Interaction and Retrieval. Association for Computing Machinery, pp. 175–184.

Ono Academic College. (2022). Roim Rachok Program. [Online] Available at: www.roim-rachok.org/english (accessed 13 August 2022).

Posar, A. and Visconti, P. (2017). Tribute to Grunya Efimovna Sukhareva, the woman who first described infantile autism. *Journal of Pediatric Neurosciences*, 12(3), pp. 300–301.

Relia, S. and Ekambaram, V. (2018). Pharmacological approach to sleep disturbances in autism spectrum disorders with psychiatric comorbidities: A literature review. *Medical Sciences*, 6(4), p. 95.

Reser, J. E. (2011). Conceptualizing the autism spectrum in terms of natural selection and behavioral ecology: The solitary forager hypothesis. *Evolutionary Psychology*, 9(2), 147470491100900209.

Sarrett, J. C. (2016). Biocertification and neurodiversity: The role and implications of self-diagnosis in autistic communities. *Neuroethics*, 9(1), pp. 23–36.

Sha, Z., Van Rooij, D., Anagnostou, E., Arango, C., Auzias, G., Behrmann, M., Bernhardt, B., Bolte, S., Busatto, G. F., Calderoni, S., and Calvo, R. (2022). Subtly altered topological asymmetry of brain structural covariance networks in autism. In: *The 28th Annual Meeting of the Organization for Human Brain Mapping* (OHBM 2022).

Sheffer, E. (2018). *Asperger's Children: The Origins of Autism in Nazi Vienna*. W. W. Norton & Company.

Sher, D. A. and Gibson, J. L. (2021). Pioneering, prodigious and perspicacious: Grunya Efimovna Sukhareva's life and contribution to conceptualising autism and schizophrenia. *European Child & Adolescent Psychiatry*, pp. 1–16.

Silberman, S. (2015). *Neurotribes: The Legacy of Autism and the Future of Neurodiversity*. Penguin.

Simmonds, C. (2019). G. E. Sukhareva's place in the history of autism research: Context, reception, translation. Doctoral dissertation at Victoria University of Wellington. [Online] Available from: http://researcharchive.vuw.ac.nz/handle/10063/8266?show=full (accessed 9 November 2022).

Ssucharewa, G. E. (1926). Die schizoiden Psychopathien im Kindesalter. *Monatsschrift für Psychiatrie und Neurologie*, 60(3–4), pp. 235–261.

State of California. (2021). California launches program to compensate survivors of state-sponsored sterilization. [Online] Available at: www.gov.ca.gov/2021/12/31/california-launches-program-to-compensate-survivors-of-state-sponsored-sterilizat ion (accessed 13 August 2022).

Stuart, N., Whitehouse, A., Palermo, R., Bothe, E., and Badcock, N. (2022). Eye Gaze in Autism Spectrum Disorder: A Review of Neural Evidence for the Eye Avoidance Hypothesis. *Journal of Autism and Developmental Disorders*, pp. 1–22.

Taylor, H., Fernandes, B., and Wraight, S. (2022). The evolution of complementary cognition: Humans cooperatively adapt and evolve through a system of collective cognitive search. *Cambridge Archaeological Journal*, 32(1), pp. 61–77.

Whatcott, J. (2020). Sexuality, disability and madness in California's eugenics era. In: R. Shuttleworth and L. Mona (eds.), *The Routledge Handbook of Disability and Sexuality*. Routledge, pp. 121–131.

Wolff, S. (2004). The history of autism. *European Child & Adolescent Psychiatry*, 13(4), pp. 201–208.

Chapter 4

Akpanglo-Nartey, J. N. and Akpanglo-Nartey, R. A. (2012). Some endangered languages of Ghana. *American Journal of Linguistics*, 1(2), pp. 10–18.

Alphabet, Inc. (2022). How search works. [Online] Available at: www.google.com/search/howsearchworks (accessed 10 September 2022).

Cohen, S. (1976). The history of the history of American education, 1900–1976: The uses of the past. *Harvard Educational Review*, 46(3), pp. 298–330.

Gross, J. A. (1980). Principles of differentiation of instruction. In: J. B. Jordan and J. A. Grassi (eds.), *An Administrator's Handbook on Designing Programs for the Gifted and Talented*. Council for Extraordinary Children, pp. 138–147.

Gutierrez-Vera, M. (2022). "Ethnic" Some Days, White the Rest: Whittier, CA as a Case Study in Mexican-American Racialization and Assimilation in Los Angeles County. *CMC Senior Theses* 3025. [Online] Available at: https://scholarship.claremont.edu/cmc_theses/3025 (accessed 9 November 2022).

Htoo, T. (2019). အော်တစ်ဇင် (Autism) မှတ်ဉာဏ်မဖွံ့ဖြိုးမှု ရောဂါ. [Online] Available at: https://yoyarlay.com/snsldfcq (accessed 7 August 2022).

Logan, J. (2022). A confusion of tongues: Trauma, fantasy, and dissociation in Lacanian theory and the imperative for social change. *Theory & Psychology*, 09593543221110824.

Lomas, R. (2011). *The Secret Power of Masonic Symbols: The Influence of Ancient Symbols on the Pivotal Moments in History and an Encyclopedia of All the Key Masonic Symbols*. Fair Winds Press.

Orfson-Offei, E. (2021). Autism spectrum disorder and language choice in Ghana. *Pragmatics and Society*, 12(2), pp. 288–308.

Pop-Jordanova, N. and Zorcec, T. (2021). Does the M-Chat-R give important information for the diagnosis of the autism spectrum disorder? *Prilozi*, 42(1), pp. 67–75.

Ramírez, L., Levy, S. R., Velilla, E., and Hughes, J. M. (2010). Considering the roles of culture and social status: The Protestant work ethic and egalitarianism. *Revista Latinoamericana de Psicologia*, 42(3), pp. 381–390.

Schwartz, T. L., Nihalani, N., Jindal, S., Virk, S., and Jones, N. (2004). Psychiatric medication-induced obesity: A review. *Obesity Reviews*, 5(2), pp. 115–121.

Wilton, R., Hansen, S., and Hall, E. (2017). Disabled people, medical inadmissibility, and the differential politics of immigration. *The Canadian Geographer/Le Géographe Canadien*, 61(3), pp. 389–400.

Yeung, J. (2021). Save the Children staff confirmed dead in Myanmar Christmas Eve attack. CNN. [Online] Available at: https://cnn.com/2021/12/28/asia/myanmar-attack-save-the-children-intl-hnk/index.html (accessed 14 August 2022).

Zeidan, J., Fombonne, E., Scorah, J., Ibrahim, A., Durkin, M. S., Saxena, S., Yusuf, A., Shih, A., and Elsabbagh, M. (2022). Global prevalence of autism: A systematic review update. *Autism Research*, 15(5), pp. 778–790.

Chapter 5

American Psychiatric Association. (2022). Diagnostic and Statistical Manual of Mental Disorders (DSM-5-TR). [Online] Available at: https://psychiatry.org/psychiatrists/practice/dsm (accessed 14 August 2022).

Atsma, A. (2017). Pyroeis. Theoi Project. [Online] Available at: www.theoi.com/Titan/AsterPyroeis.html (accessed 6 August 2022).

Carey, B. (2012). New definition of autism will exclude many, study suggests. *The New York Times*, p. 20.

Chen, Y. F. (2002). Chinese Classification of Mental Disorders (CCMD-3): Towards integration in international classification. *Psychopathology*, 35(2–3), pp. 171–175.

Clark, E. and Zhou, Z. (2005). Autism in China: From acupuncture to applied behavior analysis. *Psychology in the Schools*, 42(3), pp. 285–295.

De Blasio, F. V. (2018). *Mysteries of Mars*. Praxis.

de Broize, M., Evans, K., Whitehouse, A. J., Wray, J., Eapen, V., and Urbanowicz, A. (2022). Exploring the experience of seeking an autism diagnosis as an adult. *Autism in Adulthood*, 4(2), pp. 130–140.

Dubs, H. H. (1958). The beginnings of Chinese astronomy. *Journal of the American Oriental Society*, 78(4), pp. 295–300.

Elemy. (2022). Is autism being over diagnosed? (the status in 2022). [Online] Available at: www.elemy.com/studio/autism-diagnosis/is-it-overdiagnosed (accessed 14 August 2022).

Evans, J. (1998). *The History and Practice of Ancient Astronomy*. Oxford University Press.

FindLaw. (2016). Private special education and reimbursement FAQ. [Online] Available at: www.findlaw.com/education/spec ial-education-and-disabilities/private-special-education-and-reimbursement-faq.html (accessed 10 September 2022).

Flores-Rodríguez, Y., Ceballos, O. R., and Albores-Gallo, L. (2022). Assessing autism with DSM-IV and DSM-5 criteria using the Childhood Autism Rating Scale (CARS). *Salud Mental*, 45(1), pp. 3–10.

Flynn, A. and Polak, N. (2019). Incorporating the Power Threat Meaning Framework into an autism and learning disability team. *Clinical Psychology Forum*, 313, pp. 42–46.

Fulbrook, M. (2019). A *Concise History of Germany*. Cambridge University Press.

Gensic, J. and Brunton, J. (2022). *The #ActuallyAutistic Guide to Advocacy: Step-by-Step Advice on How to Ally and Speak Up with Autistic People and the Autism Community*. Jessica Kingsley Publishers.

Graf, F. (2015). Ares. In: T. Whitmarsh (ed.), *Oxford Research Encyclopedia of Classics*. [Online] Available at: https://oxfordre.com/classics/page/515 (accessed 6 August 2022).

Hoerricks, J. (2022). Are there two sides of the ABA coin? The AutSide. [Online] Available at: https://autside.substack.com/p/are-there-two-sides-to-the-aba-coin (accessed 18 August 2022).

Isaksen, J., Diseth, T. H., Schjølberg, S., and Skjeldal, O. H. (2013). Autism spectrum disorders–are they really epidemic? *European Journal of Paediatric Neurology*, 17(4), pp. 327–333.

Jones, A. (2006). The astronomical inscription from Keskintos, Rhodes. *Mediterranean Archaeology and Archaeometry*, 6, pp. 215–222.

Keltie, J. S. ed. (1881). *A History of the Scottish Highlands, Highland Clans and Highland Regiments*. Vol. 1. Fullarton.

Lewis, L. F. (2016). Exploring the experience of self-diagnosis of autism spectrum disorder in adults. *Archives of Psychiatric Nursing*, 30(5), pp. 575–580.

Lodi-Smith, J., Rodgers, J. D., Cunningham, S. A., Lopata, C., and Thomeer, M. L. (2019). Meta-analysis of Big Five personality traits in autism spectrum disorder. *Autism*, 23(3), pp. 556–565.

Madaus, J. W. (2008). Employment self-disclosure rates and rationales of university graduates with learning disabilities. *Journal of Learning Disabilities*, 41(4), pp. 291–299.

Masters, N. (2013). Why did a 1542 Spanish voyage refer to San Pedro Bay as the "Bay of the Smoke"? [Online] Available at: www.kcet.org/shows/lost-la/why-did-a-1542-spanish-voyage-refer-to-san-pedro-bay-as-the-bay-of-the-smoke (accessed 14 August 2022).

Mazurek, M. O., Lu, F., Symecko, H., Butter, E., Bing, N. M., Hundley, R. J., Poulsen, M., Kanne, S. M., Macklin, E. A., and Handen, B. L. (2017). A prospective study of the concordance of DSM-IV and

DSM-5 diagnostic criteria for autism spectrum disorder. *Journal of Autism and Developmental Disorders*, 47(9), pp. 2783–2794.

McPartland, J. C., Reichow, B., and Volkmar, F. R. (2012). Sensitivity and specificity of proposed DSM-5 diagnostic criteria for autism spectrum disorder. *Journal of the American Academy of Child & Adolescent Psychiatry*, 51(4), pp. 368–383.

Metcalfe, D. J. (2005). Hedera helix L. *Journal of Ecology*, 93(3), pp. 632–648.

Ming, J. (2012). Autism in China: A biosocial review. *The Columbia University Journal of Global Health*, 2(1), pp. 26–29.

Mintz, M. (2017). Evolution in the understanding of autism spectrum disorder: historical perspective. *The Indian Journal of Pediatrics*, 84(1), pp. 44–52.

Ogston, P. L., Mackintosh, V. H., and Myers, B. J. (2011). Hope and worry in mothers of children with an autism spectrum disorder or Down syndrome. *Research in Autism Spectrum Disorders*, 5(4), pp. 1378–1384.

Pellicano, E., Dinsmore, A., and Charman, T. (2014). What should autism research focus upon? Community views and priorities from the United Kingdom. *Autism*, 18(7), pp. 756–770.

Retief, M. and Letšosa, R. (2018). Models of disability: A brief overview. *HTS Teologiese Studies/Theological Studies*, 74(1).

Rice, C. E., Carpenter, L. A., Morrier, M. J., Lord, C., DiRienzo, M., Boan, A., Skowyra, C., Fusco, A., Baio, J., Esler, A., and Zahorodny, W. (2022). Defining in detail and evaluating reliability of DSM-5 criteria for Autism Spectrum Disorder (ASD) among children. *Journal of Autism and Developmental Disorders*, 52(12), pp. 1–13.

Roy, J. F. (1976). *A Guide to Barroom: The Mars of Edgar Rice Burroughs*. Ballantine Books.

Rutter, M. (1996). Autism research: Prospects and priorities. *Journal of Autism and Developmental Disorders*, 26(2), pp. 257–275.

Ssucharewa, G. E. (1926). Die schizoiden Psychopathien im Kindesalter. *Monatsschrift für Psychiatrie und Neurologie*, 60(3–4), pp. 235–261.

Telwatte, A., Anglim, J., Wynton, S. K., and Moulding, R. (2017). Workplace accommodations for employees with disabilities: A multilevel model of employer decision-making. *Rehabilitation Psychology*, 62(1), pp. 7–19.

Wang, F., Lu, L., Wang, S. B., Zhang, L., Ng, C. H., Ungvari, G. S., Cao, X. L., Lu, J. P., Hou, C. L., Jia, F. J., and Xiang, Y. T. (2018). The prevalence of autism spectrum disorders in China: A comprehensive meta-analysis. *International Journal of Biological Sciences*, 14(7), pp. 717–725.

White, E. E. (2013) [1886]. *The Elements of Pedagogy*. Book on Demand Ltd.

Wing, L., Gould, J., and Gillberg, C. (2011). Autism spectrum disorders in the DSM-V: Better or worse than the DSM-IV? *Research in Developmental Disabilities*, 32(2), pp. 768–773.

Woods, R. (2017). Exploring how the social model of disability can be re-invigorated for autism: In response to Jonathan Levitt. *Disability & Society*, 32(7), pp. 1090–1095.

Worley, J. A. and Matson, J. L. (2012). Comparing symptoms of autism spectrum disorders using the current DSM-IV-TR diagnostic criteria and the proposed DSM-V diagnostic criteria. *Research in Autism Spectrum Disorders*, 6(2), pp. 965–970.

Zolyomi, A., Jones, R., and Kaftan, T. (2020). #ActuallyAutistic sense-making on Twitter. In: T. Guerreiro, H. Nicolau, and K. Moffatt (eds.), *ASSETS '20: Proceedings of the 22nd International ACM SIGACCESS Conference on Computers and Accessibility*. Association for Computing Machinery, pp. 1–4.

Chapter 6

Ahmed, S., Sanghvi, K., and Yeo, D. (2020). Telemedicine takes centre stage during COVID-19 pandemic. *BMJ Innovations*, 6(4), pp. 252–254.

Animal Capture Wildlife Control. (2019). 5 reasons you shouldn't be afraid of opossums. [Online] Available at: www.animalcapture wildlifecontrol.com/blog/5-reasons-you-shouldnt-be-afraid-of-opossums (accessed 14 August 2022).

Ardebili, M. E., Naserbakht, M., Bernstein, C., Alazmani-Noodeh, F., Hakimi, H., and Ranjbar, H. (2021). Healthcare providers experience of working during the COVID-19 pandemic: A qualitative study. *American Journal of Infection Control*, 49(5), pp. 547–554.

Arendt, H. (1970). *On Violence*. Houghton Mifflin Harcourt.

Baochang, G., Feng, W., Zhigang, G., and Erli, Z. (2007). China's local and national fertility policies at the end of the twentieth century. *Population and Development Review*, 33(1), pp. 129–147.

Bẹwaji, J. A. I. (2018). Yorùbá values and the environment. *Yoruba Studies Review*, 3(1), pp. 1–21.

Bhatia, N. (2020). We need to talk about rationing: The need to normalize discussion about healthcare rationing in a post COVID-19 era. *Journal of Bioethical Inquiry*, 17(4), pp. 731–735.

Binkley, C. E. and Kemp, D. S. (2020). Ethical rationing of personal protective equipment to minimize moral residue during the COVID-19 pandemic. *Journal of the American College of Surgeons*, 230(6), pp. 1111–1113.

Botha, M. and Cage, E. (2022). "Autism research is in crisis": A mixed method study of researcher's constructions of autistic people and autism research. OSF Preprints. [Online] Available at: https://osf.io/w4389 (accessed 7 August 2022).

Bradshaw, C. J. and Brook, B. W. (2014). Human population reduction is not a quick fix for environmental problems.

Proceedings of the National Academy of Sciences, 111(46), pp. 16610–16615.

Chen, W. J., Zhang, Z., Wang, H., Tseng, T. S., Ma, P., and Chen, L. S. (2021). Perceptions of Autism Spectrum Disorder (ASD) etiology among parents of children with ASD. *International Journal of Environmental Research and Public Health*, 18(13), p. 6774.

Clifford, E. and Dunk, M. (2021). Disabled people's deaths don't count: How a protected characteristic offered disabled people little protection during this pandemic. In: *COVID-19 and Co-production in Health and Social Care Research, Policy, and Practice*. Policy Press, pp. 99–108.

degli Espinosa, F. (2022). Teaching generalized question-discrimination skills to children with autism: Conceptual and applied considerations. *Behavioral Interventions*, 37(1), pp. 43–55.

DuQuette, L. M. (2001). *The Chicken Qabalah of Rabbi Lamed Ben Clifford: Dilettante's Guide to What You Do and Do Not Need to Know to Become a Qabalist*. Weiser Books.

Factor, R. S., Ollendick, T. H., Cooper, L. D., Dunsmore, J. C., Rea, H. M., and Scarpa, A. (2019). All in the family: A systematic review of the effect of caregiver-administered autism spectrum disorder interventions on family functioning and relationships. *Clinical Child and Family Psychology Review*, 22(4), pp. 433–457.

Faggioni, M. P., González-Melado, F. J., and Di Pietro, M. L. (2021). National health system cuts and triage decisions during the COVID-19 pandemic in Italy and Spain: Ethical implications. *Journal of Medical Ethics*, 47(5), pp. 300–307.

Fallows, C., Gallagher, A. J., and Hammerschlag, N. (2013). White sharks (*Carcharodon carcharias*) scavenging on whales and its potential role in further shaping the ecology of an apex predator. *PloS One*, 8(4), e60797.

Fennell, L. C. and Johnson, S. A. (2022). Examination of professional biases about autism: How can we do better? *The Clinical Neuropsychologist*, 36(5), pp. 1094–1115.

Galton, F. (1904). Eugenics: Its definition, scope and aims. *American Journal of Sociology*, 10(1), pp. 1–25.

Gardner, A. L. (1982). Virginia opossum. In: J. A. Chapman and G. A. Feldhamer (eds.), *Wild Mammals of North America: Biology, Management, and Economics*. Johns Hopkins University Press, pp. 3–36.

Hancock, G. (2009). *Underworld: The Mysterious Origins of Civilization*. Crown.

Hens, K. (2019). The many meanings of autism: Conceptual and ethical reflections. *Developmental Medicine & Child Neurology*, 61(9), pp. 1025–1029.

Hoerricks, K. J. (2018). *Higher Education Support Strategies: An Evaluation of Needs Satisfaction on Autistic College Student Retention*. Doctoral dissertation. Trident University International.

Inger, R., Per, E., Cox, D. T., and Gaston, K. J. (2016). Key role in ecosystem functioning of scavengers reliant on a single common species. *Scientific Reports*, 6(1), pp. 1–5.

Jaswal, V. K. and Akhtar, N. (2019). Being versus appearing socially uninterested: Challenging assumptions about social motivation in autism. *Behavioral and Brain Sciences*, 42.

Jones, S. C. (2021). Let's talk about autistic autism researchers. *Autism in Adulthood*, 3(3), pp. 206–208.

Kavanagh, A., Hatton, C., Stancliffe, R. J., Aitken, Z., King, T., Hastings, R., Totsika, V., Llewellyn, G., and Emerson, E. (2022). Health and healthcare for people with disabilities in the UK during the COVID-19 pandemic. *Disability and Health Journal*, 15(1), 101171.

Kelly, R., O'Malley, M. P., and Antonijevic, S. (2018). "Just trying to talk to people… It's the hardest": Perspectives of adolescents with high-functioning autism spectrum disorder on their social communication skills. *Child Language Teaching and Therapy*, 34(3), pp. 319–334.

Keynes, J. M. (1926). The End of Laissez-Faire. [Online] Available at: https://panarchy.org/keynes/laissezfaire.1926.html (accessed 9 November 2022).

Knutson, S. A. (2019). The materiality of myth: Divine objects in Norse mythology. *Temenos-Nordic Journal of Comparative Religion*, 55(1), pp. 29–53.

Krueger, J. (2019). To challenge the settler colonial narrative of Native Americans in social studies curriculum. *The History Teacher*, 52(2), pp. 291–318.

Leaf, J. B., Cihon, J. H., Leaf, R., McEachin, J., Liu, N., Russell, N., Unumb, L., Shapiro, S., and Khosrowshahi, D. (2022). Concerns about ABA-based intervention: An evaluation and recommendations. *Journal of Autism and Developmental Disorders*, 52(6), pp. 2838–2853.

Lewin, N. and Akhtar, N. (2021). Neurodiversity and deficit perspectives in *The Washington Post*'s coverage of autism. *Disability & Society*, 36(5), pp. 812–833.

Lewis, L. F., Ward, C., Jarvis, N., and Cawley, E. (2021). "Straight sex is complicated enough!": The lived experiences of autistics who are gay, lesbian, bisexual, asexual, or other sexual orientations. *Journal of Autism and Developmental Disorders*, 51(7), pp. 2324–2337.

Lord, C., Brugha, T. S., Charman, T., Cusack, J., Dumas, G., Frazier, T., Jones, E. J., Jones, R. M., Pickles, A., State, M. W., and Taylor, J. L. (2020). Autism spectrum disorder. *Nature Reviews Disease Primers*, 6(1), pp. 1–23.

McDonald, T. A. M. (2020). Autism identity and the "lost generation": Structural validation of the autism spectrum identity scale and comparison of diagnosed and self-diagnosed adults on the autism spectrum. *Autism in Adulthood*, 2(1), pp. 13–23.

McRuer, D. L. and Jones, K. D. (2009). Behavioral and nutritional aspects of the Virginian opossum (*Didelphis virginiana*). *Veterinary Clinics of North America: Exotic Animal Practice*, 12(2), pp. 217–236.

Miller, D., Rees, J., and Pearson, A. (2021). "Masking is life": Experiences of masking in autistic and nonautistic adults. *Autism in Adulthood*, 3(4), pp. 330–338.

Moore, I., Morgan, G., Welham, A., and Russell, G. (2022). The intersection of autism and gender in the negotiation of identity: A systematic review and metasynthesis. *Feminism & Psychology*, 09593535221074806.

Oakley, B. F., Jones, E. J., Crawley, D., Charman, T., Buitelaar, J., Tillmann, J., Murphy, D. G., and Loth, E. (2022). Alexithymia in autism: Cross-sectional and longitudinal associations with social-communication difficulties, anxiety and depression symptoms. *Psychological Medicine*, 52(8), pp. 1458–1470.

Partington, J. S. (2003). HG Wells's eugenic thinking of the 1930s and 1940s. *Utopian Studies*, 14(1), pp. 74–81.

Reser, J. E. (2011). Conceptualizing the autism spectrum in terms of natural selection and behavioral ecology: The solitary forager hypothesis. *Evolutionary Psychology*, 9(2), 147470491100900209.

Sedgewick, F., Hull, L., and Ellis, H. (2021). *Autism and Masking: How and Why People Do It, and the Impact It Can Have*. Jessica Kingsley Publishers.

Shaw, G. B. (1910). Amazing Speech by G. B. S., Barefaced Advocacy of Free Love, Socialist Hopes. [Online] Available at: https://eugenics.us/george-bernard-shaw-and-murder-by-the-state-marriage-and-eugenics/209.htm (accessed 7 August 2022).

Shaw, G. B. (1931). Speech by George Bernard Shaw. [Online] Available at: https://youtu.be/B-Ljkoh_vmE (accessed 7 August 2022).

Sproul, B. (1979). *Primal Myths: Creation Myths Around the World*. HarperOne.

Stack, G. J. (1973). Kierkegaard: The self and ethical existence. *Ethics*, 83(2), pp. 108–125.

Stark, M. D. and Lindo, E. J. (2022). Executive functioning supports for college students with an Autism Spectrum Disorder. *Review Journal of Autism and Developmental Disorders*, pp. 1–11. [Online] Available at: https://link.springer.com/article/10.1007/s40489-022-00311-z (accessed 14 August 2022).

Stroe, M. A. (2020). Zecharia Sitchin on the Earth Chronicles: A concise lexicon of Sumerian lore. *Creativity*, 3(2), pp. 65–138.

Taggart, L., Mulhall, P., Kelly, R., Trip, H., Sullivan, B., and Wallén, E. F. (2022). Preventing, mitigating, and managing future pandemics for people with an intellectual and developmental disability – Learnings from COVID-19: A scoping review. *Journal of Policy and Practice in Intellectual Disabilities*, 19(1), pp. 4–34.

US National Park Service. (2021). Native Peoples of the Sonoran Desert: The Nde. National Park Service. [Online] Available at: https://home.nps.gov/articles/apache.htm (accessed 13 August 2022).

Webb, S. (1926). The end of laissez-faire. *Economic Journal*, 36(143), pp. 434–441.

Yang, J. M. (2019a). *The Dao De Jing: A Qigong Interpretation*. 1st ed. YMAA Publication Center.

Yang, J. M. (2019b). *The Dao in Action: Inspired Tales for Life*. 1st ed. YMAA Publication Center.

Chapter 7

Centers for Disease Control and Prevention (CDC). (2022). What is Autism Spectrum Disorder? [Online] Available at: www.cdc.gov/ncbddd/autism/facts.html (accessed 14 August 2022).

Kahn, A. (2022). Humans are not separate from nature, we're part of it. Woke Scientist Substack. [Online] Available at: https://wokescientist.substack.com/p/humans-are-not-separate-from-nature (accessed 25 August 2022).

Moon, E. (2002). *The Speed of Dark*. Warner Books UK.

Walker, N. (2021). *Neuroqueer Heresies: Notes on the Neurodiversity Paradigm, Autistic Empowerment, and Postnormal Possibilities.* Autonomous Press.

Index

www.ingramcontent.com/pod-product-compliance
Lightning Source LLC
Chambersburg PA
CBHW061249220326
41599CB00028B/5589